# Leveraging the Potential of Artificial Intelligence in the Real World

Artificial Intelligence (AI) is reshaping our urban landscapes and healthcare systems. From enhancing efficiency in smart cities to delivering personalized healthcare solutions, AI holds the key to a transformative future.

Comprising seven insightful chapters, this book offers a comprehensive overview of key topics shaping the future of healthcare systems and smart cities. This book is a combination of the smart healthcare system and the intelligent transportation system based on AI. From telemedicine's global accessibility to the application of data-mining techniques in predicting cardiac diseases and detecting anti-malaria drug resistance, each chapter presents cutting-edge research and practical applications.

Furthermore, this book explores the integration of advanced AI technologies into healthcare systems, paving the way for cost-effective solutions and innovative approaches. It also delves into the challenges associated with analyzing electroencephalogram data and predicting anxiety and depression among elderly patients, offering promising solutions and insights.

This book discusses the realms of smart cities and healthcare, where AI promises to revolutionize efficiency, sustainability, and personalized care delivery.

Researchers/scholars and graduate students at universities/research institutes and research engineers in computer science, transportation, and engineering industries will find this book beneficial.

# Leveraging the Potential of Artificial Intelligence in the Real World

## Smart Cities and Healthcare

Edited by
Tien Anh Tran, Edeh Michael Onyema, and
Arij Naser Abougreen

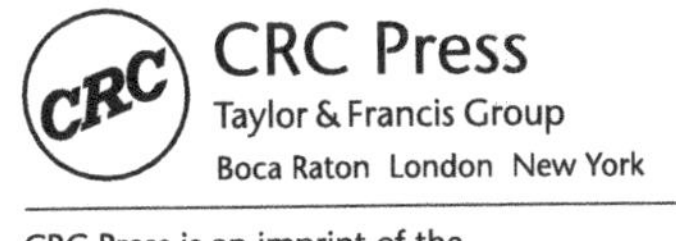

CRC Press
Taylor & Francis Group
Boca Raton  London  New York

CRC Press is an imprint of the
Taylor & Francis Group, an **informa** business

Designed cover image: © Shutterstock

First edition published 2025
by CRC Press
2385 NW Executive Center Drive, Suite 320, Boca Raton FL 33431

and by CRC Press
4 Park Square, Milton Park, Abingdon, Oxon, OX14 4RN

*CRC Press is an imprint of Taylor & Francis Group, LLC*





ISBN: 9781032667485 (hbk)
ISBN: 9781032667492 (pbk)
ISBN: 9781032667508 (ebk)

DOI: 10.1201/9781032667508

Typeset in Adobe Caslon Pro
by KnowledgeWorks Global Ltd.

# Contents

# Preface

Artificial Intelligence (AI) has the potential to revolutionize various aspects of our lives, including the functioning of cities and the delivery of healthcare services. By harnessing the power of AI, smart cities can become more efficient, sustainable, and livable, while healthcare providers can deliver more personalized, precise, and timely care to patients. Therefore, this book *Leveraging the Potential of Artificial Intelligence in the Real World: Smart Cities and Healthcare* has been written and now published by CRC Press.

In healthcare, AI has the potential to transform diagnosis, treatment planning, drug discovery, and patient monitoring. By analyzing large volumes of medical data, AI algorithms can help doctors diagnose diseases earlier and more accurately, tailor treatments to individual patients' needs, and monitor patients' health status in real-time.

The book consists of seven chapters, each of which is summarized briefly as follows:

Chapter 1 explains the concept of telemedicine, which involves the provision of general healthcare services and the remote management of medical care. Telemedicine has been shown through numerous studies to enhance patient care, reduce hospital readmission rates, and generate savings for both patients and physicians. It allows patients to be diagnosed and treated online, making healthcare more accessible globally. As healthcare professionals become more aware of its benefits, patients gain increased access to telemedicine services, and payers witness a decrease in healthcare costs. Despite its potential for growth and widespread adoption, there are various health policy implications and barriers that hinder its full utilization. Policies that support and incentivize the use and dissemination of telemedicine can help overcome these challenges.

Chapter 2 focuses on the growing concern of heart diseases in global public health, with an increasing number of cardiac patients due to unhealthy habits and insufficient health knowledge. The research aims to explore various data-mining technologies and methods applicable in the healthcare industry for accurate diagnosis and forecasting of cardiac diseases. By utilizing patient clinical data, a heart disease prediction model employing data-mining techniques can assist medical professionals in determining the patient's heart disease state. The chapter highlights the potential of machines as effective tools for data-mining categorization in healthcare, contributing to better decision-making processes. Data-mining techniques such as decision trees, Naïve Bayes, neural networks, and support vector machines (SVMs) can be effectively used in the healthcare industry to diagnose and forecast cardiac disease.

Chapter 3 assesses a range of machine learning algorithms, including K-Nearest Neighbor (KNN), Naïve Bayes, decision tree, SVM, and random forest algorithms in detecting anti-malaria drug resistance in *Plasmodium falciparum*.

Chapter 4 outlines how the integration of advanced technologies, particularly AI can revolutionize the healthcare system. It discusses various state-of-the-art techniques and methodologies applicable to healthcare, emphasizing cost-effective solutions. The chapter explores advancements in smart wearable devices and non-invasive diagnosis protocols as key components for developing cost-effective smart healthcare solutions. Integration of AI-based algorithms for analyzing vital sensor data is highlighted as crucial for adding intelligence to healthcare devices. The chapter covers innovative healthcare solutions such as digital diagnosis, ambient assisted living, social robots, remote surgeries, and virtual nurses. It addresses goals such as early diagnosis, personalized wellness, and cost feasibility for broad accessibility. The chapter also addresses current limitations of AI in healthcare and future prospects, including explainable AI and federated learning.

Chapter 5 outlines fundamental concepts of ultraviolet-induced carcinogenesis, discussing recent advancements in diagnosis and treatment. It highlights oxidative stress and reactive oxygen species as constant factors in skin cells from both external and internal sources. The chapter suggests using machine learning techniques, particularly the Hybrid Cuckoo Search Optimization with Support Vector Machine algorithm (HCSOSVM), for predicting skin illnesses. Different imaging techniques, including epiluminescence microscopy and confocal laser scan microscopy, are mentioned for diagnosis. The chapter proposes that implementing the suggested prediction method could lead to better patient outcomes. The chapter also discusses the cost-effectiveness of skin cancer prevention and early melanoma detection, highlighting their potential to improve both the economy and public health.

Chapter 6 discusses the challenges associated with analyzing electroencephalogram (EEG) data due to artifacts and proposes a real-time approach for artifact detection using Morphological Component Analysis. Specifically, the focus is on identifying eye-blink artifacts in EEG signals recorded with a TGAM EEG sensor. This research highlights the importance of artifact detection and offers a promising solution for extracting clean EEG data in real-time applications.

Chapter 7 aims to analyze research questions related to predicting anxiety and depression among elderly patients. The chapter highlights the potential benefits of using machine learning (ML) in this context for administration, health consultants, policymakers, and researchers. It explores the implications of ML in predicting anxiety and depression disorders among the elderly and emphasizes the importance of ML in diagnosing these conditions, implementing appropriate measures, and identifying potential research directions.

In conclusion, the editors wish to express their gratitude to all the contributors for generously sharing their expertise and excellent contributions, which have greatly contributed to the creation of this book.

Enjoy reading!

**Editors**
**Tien Anh Tran, Ph.D.**
**Edeh Michael Onyema, Ph.D.**
**Arij Naser Abougreen, M.Sc.**

# About the Editors

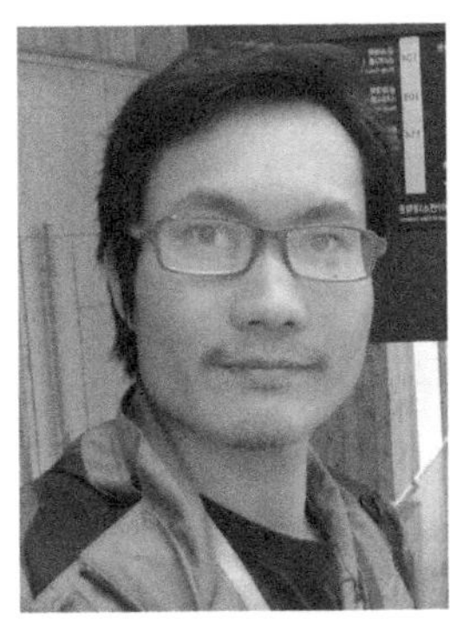

**Tien Anh Tran**
**Senior Researcher at Seoul National University, Seoul City, South Korea**
He is an Assistant Professor (Lecturer) in the Department of Marine Engineering, Vietnam Maritime University, Haiphong City, Vietnam. He is an Honorary Professor at the School of Computing Science and Engineering, Galgotias University, India and an Honorary Adjunct Professor at the School of Computer Science and Engineering, Lovely Professional University (LPU), India. Additionally, he is an Adjunct Faculty at Saveetha Institute of Medical and Technical Sciences (SIMATS) Engineering in Tamilnadu, India. He received B.Eng. and M.Sc. at Vietnam Maritime University, Vietnam in 2011 and 2014, respectively. He received a Ph.D. at Wuhan University of Technology, Wuhan, China in 2018. He is an Editor/Guest Editor for the reputation journals indexed in SCI/SCIE such as *Environment, Development and Sustainability, IET Intelligent Transport System, International Journal of Distributed Sensor Networks, Sustainable Computing: Informatics and Systems, International Journal of Renewable Energy Technology,*

*International Journal of Energy Optimization and Engineering, IEEE Internet of Things Magazine*, and *Mathematics*. In 2015, he was awarded the Chinese Government Scholarship (CSC) for the full funding of his Doctor of Philosophy (PhD) program in China. In 2019, he was awarded the NEPTUNE prize for the outstanding researchers by Vietnam Maritime University. In 2022, he was one of five outstanding scientists in Vietnam to be nominated for the ***Ta Quang Buu*** prize by the National Foundation for Science & Technology Development (NAFOSTED). Additionally, he was selected and awarded a full scholarship for the Postdoctoral Fellowship Program of the National Research Foundation (NRF) for Foreign Researchers by the Government of South Korea.

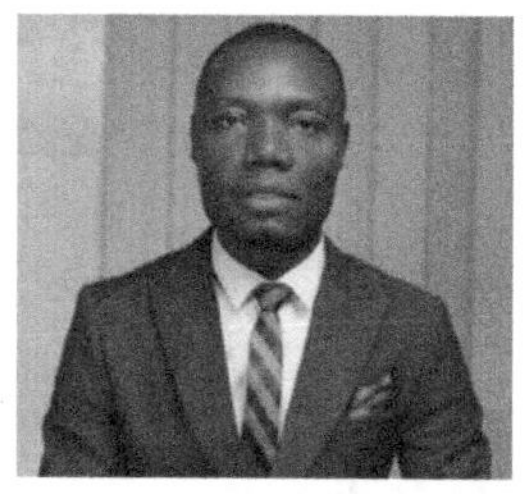

**Michael Onyema Edeh** is an Adjunct Professor at Shobhit University, India. He is currently the Head of Department, Mathematics and Computer Science at Coal City University, Nigeria. Michael is a Recipient of the prestigious Chancellor's Award for Best Staff of the Year 2020, and Vice Chancellor's Award for research Excellence 2023, both at Coal City University. He is also the current Chairman of the Nigeria Computer Society (NCS), Enugu State Chapter, Nigeria. Michael has taught Computer Science courses to both postgraduate and undergraduate students in several tertiary education institutions, including Southwestern University; Coal City University; Spiritan University Nneochi; National Open University of Nigeria (NOUN); Alex Ekwueme Federal University Ebonyi State; Gregory University Uturu; Enugu State College of Education Technical affiliated to Nnamdi Azikiwe University Nigeria; Institute of Management and Technology (IMT) Enugu; African Thinkers Community of Inquiry College of Education (ATCOI-COE) Enugu; Pogil College of Health Technology Ogun State; and Federal Science and Technical College Ogun State. He has published more than 100 scholarly papers in reputable journals, and also acted as an editor and reviewer for many top journals. He has interest in cybersecurity, education, machine learning and cloud computing.

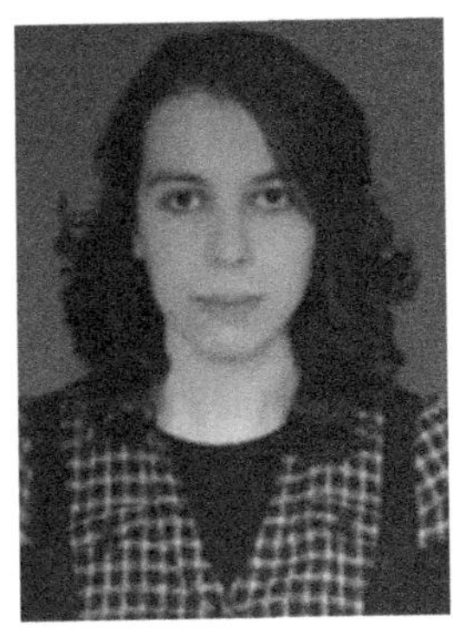

**Arij Naser Abougreen** received the M.Sc. degree in Communication Engineering from the University of Tripoli, Libya, in 2018. She is a Ph.D. student at Istanbul Medipol University. Her research interests include image processing, machine learning, Internet of Things, and wireless communication. She has three years of teaching experience in reputed universities and high institutes. She served as a session chair of International Conference on Digital Technologies and Applications (ICDTA 2023) and a session chair of the International Conference on Artificial Intelligence in Information and Communication (ICAIIC 2023). Also, she served as a technical Program Committee member and a reviewer for several conferences such as **7th** IEEE World Forum on the Internet of Things (WFIoT 2021), New Orleans, USA; **11th** series of IEEE Symposium on Computer Applications and Industrial Electronics (ISCAIE 2021); **44th** International Conference on Telecommunications and Signal Processing (TSP 2021); **30th** International Conference on Computing and Communication Networks (ICCCN 2021), organized by Manchester Metropolitan University, United Kingdom; IEEE International Conference on Electronics Circuits and Systems (ICECS 2022); EAI CICom 2022; 3rd EAI International Conference on Computational Intelligence and Communications and EAI IoTaaS 2022; and the 8th EAI International Conference on IoT as a Service. She also served as a reviewer for the journal *Multimedia Tools and Applications* (Springer), *Journal of Healthcare Engineering* (Hindawi) and *Applied Artificial Intelligence* (Taylor & Francis). In addition, she served as a reviewer for IGI and Springer books. She has authored/co-authored four book chapters and two papers. She has edited a book that has been published by IGI Global. She is currently editing three books to be published by IGI Global, CRC Press, and Springer. She is also a member of IEEE Public Safety Technology Smart Algorithm and Informatics Committee.

# Contributors


**M. Banerjee**
RKDF University
Ranchi, India

**Satyabrat Malla Bujar Baruah**
Department of Electronics and
 Communication Engineering,
 Tezpur University
Napam, Sonitpur, Tezpur, India

**Kunal Biswas**
Sathyabama Institute of Science
 and Technology
Chennai, India

**Bidyut Bikash Borah**
Department of Electronics and
 Communication Engineering,
 Tezpur University
Tezpur, India

**Rakshi Anuja Dinesh**
Sathyabama Institute of Science
 and Technology
Chennai, India

**P. Divyashree**
Indian Institute of Information
 Technology
Sri City, India

**Priyanka Dwivedi**
Indian Institute of Information
 Technology
Sri City, India

**Uddipan Hazarika**
Department of Electronics and
 Communication Engineering,
 Tezpur University
Tezpur, India

**Sivanantham K**
Crapersoft
Coimbatore, India

**N. Kumari**
RKDF University
Ranchi, India

**Lailil Muflikhah**
Faculty of Computer Science,
 Brawijaya University
Malang, Indonesia

**Blessington Praveen P**
Crapersoft
Coimbatore, India

**Gayatri Panda**
NIST Institute of Science and
 Technology (Autonomous)
Berhampur, India

**Soumik Roy**
Department of Electronics and
 Communication Engineering,
 Tezpur University
Tezpur, India

**Achintya Kr. Sarkar**
Indian Institute of Information
 Technology
Sri City, India

**Jayashree Shanmugam**
Sathyabama Institute of Science
 and Technology
Chennai, India

1

# Telemedicine

## A New Horizon in Public Health Management

N. KUMARI AND M. BANERJEE

### 1.1 Introduction

Telemedicine is the delivery of medical care through the use of technology. A patient in one location can be treated by a doctor in another location via telecommunication. The medical field has adopted the usage of computers and smartphones. Videoconferencing is used for the majority of telemedicine, while care through email or the phone is preferred by certain medical professionals.

The delivery of medical services such as examinations and consultations over the Internet and other forms of telecommunication infrastructure is an example of telemedicine, which is also known as telehealth or e-medicine. Utilising the patient's own device or a telehealth kiosk, medical professionals are able to remotely examine, diagnose, and treat patients through the use of telemedicine. A home telemedicine exam often consists of the patient downloading an app such as Live Health or calling a telemedicine number that is typically offered by a primary care physician or employer as part of the health benefits package.

The remote patient will first be asked about their medical history and symptoms, and then they will be linked to a clinician. The clinician might recommend that the patient take an over-the-counter drug, get a prescription filled, go to the hospital, or make a follow-up appointment. The word "distance" comes from the Greek *tele*, while "to heal" comes from the Latin *medicare*. Telemedicine was referred to as "healing by wire" by *Time* magazine. Despite its "futuristic" and "experimental" beginnings, telemedicine is now considered a standard form of medical care.

There are several applications for telemedicine, including patient care and education, research and administration, and public health (1). People living in rural and distant areas across the world have a difficult

DOI: 10.1201/9781032667508-1

**1**

time accessing timely and high-quality medical care. Residents in suburban and rural locations frequently have limited access to specialty medical treatment as a result of the concentration of specialist physicians in urban areas. Telemedicine makes it possible for residents of rural locations to receive medical care (2, 3). Historical underpinnings:

Telemedicine has been around for more than a century. Telehealth and telemedicine have evolved alongside communication and information technologies. Medical professionals quickly recognised the potential of new technologies and sought to use them to improve healthcare delivery.

Healthcare providers know telemedicine as remote care delivery. Telehealth is growing in popularity because it fits the latest digital health trends for patient care. Telehealth refers to service delivery, while telemedicine involves using any technology in clinical settings. Most professionals use these terms interchangeably. We use the terms interchangeably as we study telemedicine's history.

## 1.2  When Did Telemedicine Begin?

A combination of the Latin word *medicus* with the Greek word *tele*, the word "telemedicine," coined by Thomas Bird in 1970, refers to "healing at a distance." The development of the telegraph and the telephone marked the beginning of telemedicine. Signal flags were used by medical personnel to alert ships to the presence of infectious diseases. These gadgets were not data transmitters for medical purposes; rather, they were extensions of human messengers. The telegraph and the telephone were the foundations upon which telemedicine was built. In spite of the telegraph requiring certain technical prerequisites, these two technologies made it possible for anybody to deliver messages or converse across great distances. After first employing telegraphs and telephones for the purpose of providing medical care, the military eventually expanded their use of these technologies to include everyday communication.

## 1.3  The Early Days of Telemedicine—Telephone and Telegraph

The telegraph was a revolutionary technology that completely altered the face of combat. During the time of the American Civil War, electronic information was used for the first time in the United States for the purpose of providing medical care. In addition to making strategic planning easier, the telegraph enabled the Union Army to do the following: Place orders for medical supplies and inform others on the battlefield of any injuries.

### 1.3.1 Report Casualties

Robert H. Eikelboom presents proof in his book *The Telegraph and the Beginnings of Telemedicine in Australia,* that the telegraph was used in Australia in 1874 to assist injured patients. This information can be found in the chapter titled "The Beginnings of Telemedicine in Australia." Alexander Graham Bell came up with the idea for the telephone in 1876. In that era, people's lives were fundamentally altered by the introduction of phones; today, however, we tend to take them for granted. Applications in the medical field for the telephone appeared rather soon. In 1879, an article published in the journal *The Lancet* discussed the possibilities of the telephone in the medical field. A doctor will listen to a baby's cough through a phone receiver to identify croup in the infant. The 20th century was a pivotal time in the development of telemedicine. The telephone network rapidly grew as the signal quality continued to improve.

The home devices now have their own individual phone numbers. The 1900s saw the widespread adoption of telephone use.

### 1.3.2 How Did This Change Affect Healthcare Delivery?

In the 20th century, telemedicine developed and flourished.

### 1.3.3 1905: Heart Sound Transmission

In 1905, Willem Einthoven transmitted heart sounds from a hospital to his laboratory using the telephone.

### 1.3.4 1910: Electrocardiography and Remote Diagnosis

New York cardiologists published the first American electrocardiography review in 1910. Cable transmission of electrocardiograms (ECGs) from the wards to the ECG room was reported. The same year, English engineer Sidney Brown modified the telephone to allow doctors to listen to a patient's stethoscope from miles away and make an accurate diagnosis.

### 1.3.5　*The 1920s: Two-Way Radio Communication*

The Haukeland Hospital in Norway started using two-way radio in 1920 so that doctors could communicate with ships and better treat sailors. During the subsequent ten years, a number of nations began implementing two-way radio communication. In 1923, Victoria, Australia, police began using mobile two-way radios to report injuries and communicate with colleagues.

### 1.3.6　*1924: A Prediction for Telemedicine as We Know It Today*

*Radio News* was the first to come up with the idea of telemedicine in April 1924. The magazine called the way patients and doctors talked through TV and microphones "radio doctor." Most Americans didn't have TVs yet, but *Radio News* showed a person receiving medical care through the TV. The magazine's first prediction that two-way video communication would be used to deliver care remotely shed light on the future of telemedicine. While there isn't much a doctor can do over the phone, with two-way video, they could treat people with conditions that needed a physical exam. Technology had to evolve before doctors and patients could video chat. This prediction came true because the telecommunication infrastructure could be scaled up for large-scale telemedicine projects.

### 1.3.7　*1959: The First Use of Two-Way Video Communication for Telemedicine Occurs*

The 1950s saw the introduction of telemedicine's first two-way video communication systems. The University of Nebraska was the first institution in the United States to implement a two-way video telemedicine system. In 1959, medical students were given neurological examinations with the use of interactive video. It was the first technology to provide real-time video communication in telemedicine. Academic institutions made use of telemedicine to facilitate the transmission of medical data such as X-rays, ECGs, stethoscope sounds, and so on.

### 1.3.8 The 1960s: Wide Adoption of Telemedicine in the United States

Telemedicine breakthrough in the 1960s included NASA, Lockheed, and the Indian Health Service initiating a massive telemedicine initiative. The Space Technology Applied to Rural Papago Advanced Health Care (STARPAHC) project made use of NASA astronaut communications to increase access to healthcare on American Indian reservations.

That era also saw the expansion of satellite communication in telemedicine and rural healthcare delivery. In 1972, the Applications Technology Satellite (ATS-1) enabled Alaska's smaller villages and hospitals with telecommunications.

After STARPHAC's success and the development of satellite communications, telemedicine grew significantly.

### 1.3.9 The 1980s: Radiology as the First Medical Specialty to Fully Embrace Telemedicine

The success of STARPHAC sparked a number of other government-funded telemedicine initiatives and projects.

The main uses of telemedicine in the 1970s and '1980s included:

- Providing medical attention to patients in conflict zones.
- Providing medical care to Arctic and Antarctic research sites.
- Providing healthcare services to inmates at correctional facilities without having to bring them to a hospital.
- Transmitting radiological pictures; radiology pioneered telemedicine in the 1980s.

Grant-funded projects helped radiologists demonstrate the efficiency and benefits of remote care, boosting telemedicine adoption. Radiologists used telemedicine more than other doctors. Telemedicine consultation images were received via technology. And with the Internet, telemedicine and telehealth history grew exponentially into what we know today.

### 1.4 The Internet Transforms Telehealth in More Ways than One

The Internet had an impact on telemedicine in the 1980s. TCP/IP, the Internet protocol suite, was adopted by the Advanced Research Projects Agency Network (ARPANET), a pioneering packet-switching network, in 1983. Bright minds from all around the world began constructing the "network of networks" that would eventually become the Internet as a result of the recently found technology. The foundation of the Internet was TCP/IP. Tim Berners-Lee created the World Wide Web seven years later, in 1990. Online data was accessible to all countries through websites and links.

The ease with which medical data and live video may be transmitted over the Internet has tremendously benefited the widespread acceptance of telemedicine. Due to the equipment's limitations, cost, and need for considerable training, even the most successful telemedicine initiatives didn't last in the 1990s. The delivery of remote healthcare was made easier and less expensive via the Internet. It improved telemedicine services by introducing new techniques for transmitting data over large distances.

***The Internet allows doctors to accomplish the following:***

- Transfer large data files at incredible speeds.
- Acquire the necessary equipment for telemedicine at much lower costs.
- Connect with their remote patients more easily.

The power of the Internet was quickly apparent and this helped in accelerating the development of its infrastructure. The Internet immediately delivered vast amounts of information. People learnt more about health challenges and their healthcare options as they acknowledged the Internet's role in health technology. Early Internet connections were excruciatingly slow. Dial-up Internet requires a phone connection and took an inordinate amount of time to load a website. As the number of Internet users increased, so did the need for faster speeds, more reliable connections, and lower rates. Healthcare distribution pioneered innovative methods of transmitting data over great distances, boosting telemedicine services.

*As a result, a variety of improvements happened, including:*

- A quicker rate of communication.
- A greater availability.
- An improvement in information storage.
- Standardisation of formats for the transfer of data.
- An increase in data security.
- An upgrade in equipment.

Broadband Internet has contributed to an expansion in telemedicine and telehealth by making it simpler for patients and physicians to participate in virtual appointments. When conducting remote patient examinations and providing real-time telemedicine services, medical professionals utilise wearable gadgets and digital cameras. Electronic medical records (EMRs) can also be created online, which makes healthcare administration much easier. It is possible that the COVID-19 pandemic had the most significant influence on the rapid rise of telemedicine in the United States.

## 1.5 Ever-changing Scenario: Now and Later

In comparison to outdated telemedicine equipment, modern telehealth gadgets are more feature-packed and take up less space. Patients' critical data can be monitored in real time using wearable technology such as fitness bracelets and heart rate monitors. The use of smart glasses and watches, which are now rather popular in the medical field, will soon be able to assist physicians with their paperwork. To automatically transcribe patient records during examinations, the digital health business Augmedix, which was created by Pelu Tran and Ian Shakil while they were medical students at Stanford, employs Google Glass. Concepts similar to this will eventually become widespread, much like telemedicine did in 1924. It is to the benefit of the telemedicine industry that there are many untapped regions. Because of the significant investment made in it by both private companies and public research organisations, telemedicine technology is advancing at a rate that is outpacing the ability of physicians to keep up.

## 1.6 Definitions and Concepts

The World Health Organization (WHO) defines telemedicine as "the delivery of healthcare services where distance is a key factor, by all healthcare professionals using information and communication technologies for the exchange of valid information for diagnosis, treatment, and prevention of disease and injuries, research and evaluation, and continuing education of healthcare providers, all with the goal of improving the health of individuals (4)." Telemedicine Consulting Centres can scan, convert, change, and send medical information about a patient. The expert is at the Telemedicine Specialty Centre (TSC) who can talk to the patient from far away and see his reports and progress.

### 1.6.1 Telemedicine System

For information exchange and teleconsultations, telemedicine uses hardware, software, and a way to talk to connect two different places through the use of computers, printers, scanners, equipment for video-conferencing, and so on. Software receives information about patients (images, reports, films etc.) and the channels of communication link the two places together.

## 1.7 Utility of Telemedicine

Simple remote access, home care, ambulatory care, critical care, continuing medical education, clinical research, public awareness, disaster management, second views, and difficult diagnoses can all be monitored using telemedicine. Once telecommunication is established, telemedicine's biggest potential is to add knowledge to medical practices, including tele-mentored procedures such as hand-controlled robot surgery and disease surveillance and programme tracking. It enables healthcare standardisation and equity across countries and continents. According to the Center for International Rehabilitation, telemedicine and telecommunications are critical to remote rehabilitation services. Telemedicine cannot replace physicians in remote locations, especially in developing nations where resources are scarce and there are numerous public health challenges. As a result, this technology cannot currently replace doctors. However, it has the potential to significantly improve health in the majority of countries.

## 1.8 Types of Technology

Most telemedicine applications use two types of technology. The first, store-and-forward, moves digital images. Using a digital camera, a computer "stores" and "forwards" a digital image. This is used in non-emergency situations when a diagnosis or consultation can be made in 24–48 hours and sent back. Teledermatology, teleradiology, and telepathology are examples (5). When a "face-to-face" consultation is needed, two-way interactive television (IATV) is used. At the originating site are the patient, provider, nurse practitioner, or telemedicine coordinator. The specialist is located at the referral site, usually an urban medical centre. Both locations have videoconferencing equipment for "real-time" consultations (6). Psychiatry, internal medicine, rehabilitation, cardiology, paediatrics, obstetrics and gynaecology, and neurology are all suitable for this type of consultation (6).

### 1.8.1 Types of Telemedicine

The three most common forms of telemedicine are known as store-and-forward, remote monitoring, and real-time interactive services. When used appropriately, each component of healthcare plays an important part in providing benefits to patients as well as those who work in the medical field.

*1.8.1.1 Store-and-forward* Telemedicine reduces patient visits. The specialist can instead receive patient photos or biosignals in specialties such as dermatology, radiology, and pathology. Store-and-forward telemedicine saves time and helps doctors provide better treatment. Using a history report and photographs instead of a physical exam can lead to misdiagnosis.

*1.8.1.2 Remote Monitoring* Remote monitoring uses gadgets to remotely monitor a patient's health and clinical symptoms. This manages diabetes, asthma, and cardiovascular diseases. Cost-effective, regular remote monitoring increases patient satisfaction. Self-tests may be erroneous, although results are similar to professional-patient exams.

*1.8.1.3 Real-time Interactive Services*   Interactive services can help patients immediately. These include phone, online, and home visits during which medical history, symptom consultation, and assessment can be done.

*1.8.1.4 Tele-neuropsychology*   Through the use of tele-neuropsychology, patients suffering from cognitive disorders can receive neuropsychological counselling and testing over the phone. The patient is examined with the use of the typical methods on video. According to the findings of a study that was conducted in 2014, this particular application of telemedicine is a practicable and trustworthy substitute for traditional face-to-face consultations; however, quality standards and administration must be maintained.

*1.8.1.5 Telenursing*   Telehealth, often known as telenursing, refers to the practise of providing medical care remotely by utilising various forms of electronic communication. Telephone consultations help detect health problems and keep track of their progression. Patients living in more remote areas are increasingly turning to this form of telemedicine since it is convenient and relatively inexpensive. By treating patients for mild ailments sooner and providing patients with advice regarding hospital admission, it is also possible to lessen the strain that patients place on hospitals.

*1.8.1.6 Tele-pharmacy*   Patients are given advice via tele-pharmacy in the event that there is no pharmacist accessible. It is possible to receive phone guidance and monitor your medication. Patients are eligible to acquire refill authorisation so that they can continue to receive their routine prescriptions.

*1.8.1.7 Telerehabilitation*   Telerehabilitation is the process of evaluating and treating rehabilitation patients through the use of technology. The ability to communicate symptoms and clinical progress more easily thanks to webcams and video conferences.

### 1.8.2 Growing Role of Artificial Intelligence in Telemedicine

Because of technological advancements, artificial intelligence (AI) is now widely used. The field of healthcare is undergoing fast changes. One of the most recent businesses to make considerable use of AI is telehealth, which includes the usage of electronic healthcare cards as well as counselling. AI has a significant impact on telemedicine in the United States. AI in telehealth enables physicians to make real-time, data-driven decisions, which in turn improves both the patient experience and the health outcomes. This is happening as practitioners increase virtual care options across the care continuum.

*1.8.2.1 Providing a More Accurate Diagnosis* Using telemedicine, remote diagnosis is feasible. Now, physicians may diagnose and cure diseases remotely. Patients with diabetic retinopathy have had fewer visits as a result. The Los Angeles County Department of Health Services discovered that diabetic retinopathy telehealth monitoring reduced patient visits by 14,000. The inclusion of AI to the screening processes is anticipated to significantly reduce the number of visits. If an AI system is utilised for screening, only retinal images will be required by the algorithm. By comparing images to previous samples, the AI system can reliably determine illness severity. Utilising AI in screening will save time and effort for physicians and patients. Another company (The Deeper Insights company) is developing an AI method to identify rare genetic abnormalities from patient photographs. Typically, seven office visits on average are required to detect uncommon genetic illnesses; telemedicine and AI can eliminate some of these office visits. The clinician can send an image of the patient's face to the AI system for diagnosis. Due to AI's ease of recognition in telemedicine, doctors and patients may anticipate faster and less expensive treatment.

*1.8.2.2 Keeping Doctors from Burning Out* During extended workdays, physicians may experience anxiety. It may result in weariness, discontent, and poor work habits. Burnout is typically triggered by extensive patient contact or technology use. AI can also help recognise indicators of exhaustion. It can even estimate a doctor's maximum patient load.

*1.8.2.3 Providing Elderly Patients with Better Medical Care*     Telemedicine apps for mobile devices assist users in managing their medical conditions, fitness goals, doctor appointments, and insurance claims. Telemedicine will employ assistive robots.

These robots will provide healthcare to residents, especially the elderly. Smart robots can help with mobility, medication delivery, and emergency alerting.

The robots can conduct their tasks semi-autonomously. AI enables robots to comprehend their environment, the patient's behaviour, and the interior of the home. As a result, it may increase patient care and assistance. The Japanese government is researching AI robots for the elderly. These robots can assist individuals with bathing, moving, disposing of waste, and checking their health in real time. These robots can provide healthcare at the same cost as people. They may improve patients' quality of life by offering 24-hour care for the elderly.

*1.8.2.4 Patient-Monitoring Convenience*     AI allows remote patient monitoring and doctor-patient simulations. The NextDREAM Consortium Group studied remote diabetes care with AI. The main finding was that remote insulin adjustments using the trialled automated AI system may be as effective as expert physician dosage changes. Doctors and specialists can use the AI-based decision support service. The University of San Francisco Center for Telehealth Innovation is testing AI to detect pneumothorax in X-rays. Telehealth AI uses include data analysis, remote patient monitoring, and intelligent diagnosis and support. AI can help doctors diagnose and treat patients, reduce burnout, and improve patient experiences. AI and telehealth are helping healthcare executives stay competitive by simplifying clinician processes and unlocking predictive potential from patient data analysis. Lockdown measures reduced the need for in-person consultations in 2024. AI has greatly improved home client monitoring

*1.8.2.5 Making Hospital Visits Easier*     Telemedicine reduces hospital visits, but some visits are necessary. In such cases, AI may help reduce patient wait times and expedite care. AI technology informs hospital staff about patient inflow, high-priority cases, bed shortages, and other patient-care issues. The programme increased the hospital's ability to treat complex patients by 60%. Ambulances are sent an hour earlier, improving efficiency. AI and predictive analytics help emergency department patients receive beds 30% faster. As telemedicine and telehealth gain popularity, AI will become increasingly important. Telehealth AI may also benefit doctors. By decreasing patient wait times, recommending the best treatment options, and making healthcare accessible 24/7, it will reduce costs, improve healthcare, and improve the workplace.

## 1.9 Challenges in Implementation

The high cost of telemedicine is a key impediment to its widespread use. Cost-effective models must be installed and trained in hospitals and facilities, which will take time and money (2). Infrastructure upgrades may be required to transmit quality telemedicine information promptly and reliably, which can be problematic in remote or underdeveloped institutions (3). Because of current concerns about confidentiality and security in telemedicine consultation and operations, AI has a promising future in healthcare information. Satellites and the Internet pose security and confidentiality risks. It may take time for studies addressing this issue to be implemented into telemedicine technology. Due to malpractice concerns, telemedicine gadgets, like other medical devices, necessitate training and licencing. This may deter facilities from deploying these technologies because it adds expense and time to the process. Malpractice and a lack of education can also have an impact on patient consistency and preference, leading to a disregard for the use or advancement of technology.

## 1.10 Advantages and Disadvantages of Telemedicine

Telemedicine is a new way to provide healthcare over long distances that uses communication and information technology. Even though this idea started in the 20th century with the telephone and radio, new technologies like the video telephone, the latest tele-medical devices, mobile cooperation technology, diagnostic methods, distributed client or server applications, etc., have improved the quality and range of telemedicine services. This system removes distance barriers in clinical healthcare. Here are the main pros and cons of telemedicine:

*Pros:*

- A lot of people dread going to the hospital or seeing their doctor. This approach makes it easier for patients and providers to communicate with one another. The transmission of medical information and photos via telemedicine is secure. As a result, it is possible to rely on and benefit from using this system. In emergencies, it saves lives. In post-disaster areas, rural areas, and isolated locations, there is a shortage of consistent healthcare. In these types of situations, emergency care can be provided using telemedicine.
- Patients in rural or outlying places can benefit from telemedicine. Clinical treatment can be administered in the patient's own home. Mobile collaboration enables medical practitioners located in different parts of the country to effortlessly communicate and discuss important patient cases with one another.
- The use of a computer, tablet, or phone for medical purposes has resulted in fewer outpatient visits. Prescriptions may be checked for accuracy and doctors can monitor drug control. Patients who are unable to leave their homes can still receive medical attention. The costs of healthcare have come down.
- This technique contributes to health education by enabling primary healthcare providers to observe experts in their professions and enabling experts to oversee novices in their respective fields.
- Telemedicine eliminates patient-provider disease transmission.

*Cons:*

- Telecom systems, especially data management equipment and medical professional training, are expensive.
- Virtual clinical treatment reduces human interaction between healthcare professionals and patients, which increases clinical error risk if provided by inexperienced professionals.
- Due to Internet speed or server issues, telemedicine may take longer. This system cannot immediately administer antibiotics.

- Poor health informatics records like X-rays, clinical progress reports, etc., can lead to poor clinical treatment.
- Telemedicine service providers need strict legal regulation to avoid unauthorised or illegal services.

## 1.11 Telemedicine Concerns and Strategy to Overcome

From 2017 to 2023, telemedicine is expected to grow 16.8%. Due to its cost savings and ease of use, more than 50% of US hospitals and 1 million Americans use it. Telemedicine has many advantages, but it also has drawbacks. Having a plan can help you overcome these concerns. Telemedicine concerns and solutions are listed here.

### 1.11.1 Reimbursement

Telemedicine reimbursement is difficult for doctors and other healthcare providers. Medicare reimburses telemedicine with restrictions.

The Medicare Chronic Management Program (United States) reimburses services for patients with two or more chronic conditions. Reimbursement claims must last at least one year or until death.

However, the Centers for Medicare and Medicaid Services (CMS) is proposing coverage for 2019 and 2024, including extended preventative services and virtual check-ins. Private insurance companies may not cover telemedicine services.

Using technology to track reimbursement claims helps overcome reimbursement challenges. A platform that tracks these expenses can help you document payer-required receipts and stay current on insurers' allowable reimbursements.

### 1.11.2 Lack of Integration

If your EHR system doesn't work with your telemedicine platform, your workflow records will likely be complicated.

You can record your workflow and ensure that your patients' televisits are properly documented and updated by using a platform that integrates with your EHR.

### 1.11.3 Lack of Sufficient Data for Care Continuity

Platform integration issues can also disrupt care. If a patient receives telemedicine from one provider but chooses another for his next televisit, the second physician may not have all the information she needs to diagnose the patient. The best option is to ask where your patient received telemedicine services, including those from hospitals and other medical facilities.

### 1.11.4 Service Awareness

Your patients won't use telemedicine if they don't know about it. It's a missed opportunity if your patients don't know you offer telemedicine services, as 96% of large employers plan to do so. Thus, content and social media marketing should be used to promote your launch via social media, email newsletters, and your blog, if you have one.

### 1.11.5 Patients' Lack of Technical Skills

Patients who don't know how to use telemedicine services can have reduce usage and accessibility. Before launching your telemedicine services, ask patients which devices they prefer to use.

It's crucial to train your staff to use telemedicine equipment so they can assist patients.

### 1.11.6 Expensive Technology

Physicians, hospitals, and medical practises may worry about telemedicine costs when they add up equipment and service costs. While telemedicine use grows, technology costs and service costs will decrease, so opting for bundled or flat-fee services may help you save.

Telemedicine is also helping patients save money on in-person visits and emergency room (ER) visits, potentially saving 25% on ER staff costs.

### 1.11.7 Privacy Concerns

While accessing patient data online, telemedicine services can pose security and privacy risks. Telemedicine services must encrypt data and network connections to comply with the Health Insurance Portability and Accountability Act (HIPAA). Patients must be messaged securely. Before recording and storing video calls, get patient consent.

## 1.12 Future of Telemedicine and Further Scope of AI Implementations

- Technology has made our dreams come true. Telemedicine is the use of communications to diagnose and treat patients from a distance. Telemedicine is on the rise, using the Internet to connect patients and doctors. E-health, m-health, and tele-health are all synonyms for telemedicine, which uses technology to connect patients and caregivers.
- Although telemedicine is a well-established service, its popularity has yet to blossom. There is more space for innovation in the industry.

### 1.12.1 What Is the Future of Telemedicine?

It's unclear, but like with every revolutionary healthcare invention, acceptance by the medical community will require time and the appropriate spark. Telemedicine has developed dramatically since February 2020. Because of the COVID-19 pandemic, telemedicine will:

- **Become a Standard Service.** Today's patients are used to telemedicine's accessibility. Over the past decade, telemedicine has steadily grown and become a key and disruptive element, not only technologically but also socioculturally and economically, because it solves current problems. Demand for health services, population ageing, and information management are these challenges.
- **Form Medical Services in Remote Locations to Connected Health.** New technologies aid in the growth of telemedicine and the implementation of globality and interoperability in healthcare organisations. Beyond telemedicine, it fosters organised work conditions for healthcare services, particularly in rural places. Telemedicine will now be able to deliver health services in remote locations while also bringing a multidisciplinary approach to primary care.

- **Make Remote Patient Care a Reality.** The provision of remote medical services by remote professionals is one of telemedicine's most prevalent applications. In the majority of nations, physicians are concentrated in a single region, forcing patients in rural places to travel great distances to receive care. By permitting remote consultations with the referral hospital, telemedicine will cut wait times for diagnosis and treatment as well as referrals in primary care. Initially, telemedicine was utilised more in the care process; however, it is currently utilised for remote patient monitoring and follow-up specifically:
  - **Teleconsultation:** Remote monitoring, diagnosis, and treatment help patients. However, clinical information must be shared. Services in this category include the transmission of x-rays or similar images (teleradiology), laboratory or electronic health record, and its application in specialities such as dermatology, psychiatry, or cardiology, among others.
  - **Telemonitoring:** It will enable the biological, physiological, and biometric monitoring of patients, typically chronic patients. Through telemonitoring, patients can be aided. Telemonitoring enables patients to engage in their care while minimising their hospital stays.
  - **Tele-Surgery:** Telesurgery is one of the biggest advances in telemedicine and will continue to improve. Robotics and virtual reality have increased experimental telesurgeries in recent years.

### *Distance Education and Decision Support for Health Professionals*

- Telemedicine has helped health systems address socio-economic issues. Telemedicine optimises health resources, improves demand management, reduces hospital stays and trips, and improves health system efficiency and sustainability.
- Telemedicine facilitates communication and collaboration between health professionals in the same city, country, or worldwide. It benefits patients and health professionals. Telemedicine has helped patients manage their illnesses and get expert help quickly. Additionally, it:
  - Brings equity in access to health services.
  - Allows collaboration between teams of clinical professionals.

- Promotes the continuity of care.
- Improves the efficiency of health services.

The COVID-19 pandemic was combated in part using telemedicine. Moreover, it has enhanced care delivery in general. Telemedicine connects remote specialists for emergency assistance, safeguards healthcare professionals from pathogens, and enables continuity of treatment for chronically ill patients. Providers, health administrators, and patients have acknowledged telemedicine's ease, quality, and innovation. Telemedicine enables health teams to expedite routine exams, continue patient monitoring, and provide more face-to-face care where it's needed. Telemedicine will employ real-time analytics to diagnose, respond to medical emergencies, and communicate information as AI and edge computing continue to advance. Intel, an American multinational corporation, is collaborating with health ecosystem hardware and software developers to scale telemedicine technology in the future.

## 1.13 Conclusions

Access to medical treatment can be improved for patients through the use of telemedicine services, particularly for those living in rural locations. Telemedicine is less expensive than in-person consultations and appointments.

An unexplored market in telemedicine is the virtual management of chronic diseases. Patients who have such concerns are required to visit the doctor on a regular basis. The use of telemedicine may result in fewer trips to the emergency room and hospital admissions. Patients who are stable but otherwise fit the requirements for hospitalisation are treated using the "hospital at home" concept. They are treated at home for chronic obstructive pulmonary disease, pneumonia, and heart failure. Even in this context, telemedicine can be helpful.

There will be a significant need for more intelligent and superior medical treatment. We need telemedicine and robotic treatments to develop and deploy current healthcare solutions in a variety of areas as medical professionals make new discoveries. Naturally, this will result in a decrease in the amount of work that is done by professionals and an increase in the demand for expertise in the maintenance of

AI- and robot-powered programmes. If AI technology is used everywhere, hospitals will be able to give care around the clock. AI and robotics might be able to aid telemedicine services during a public health emergency or outbreak while simultaneously reducing exposure to healthcare staff and systems. The AI-assisted telemedicine framework that is currently being developed by the consortium (The Deeper Insights company) may make telemedicine more accessible and facilitate its expansion into new medical fields and locations. It is possible that an international collaborative effort led by WHO, the present consortium, or other organisations of a similar nature might improve the penetration of telemedicine, particularly for the disadvantaged and those who live in low-resource situations.

# References


1. Neurosurgeon Ganapathy K., Apollo Hospitals, Chennai, Telemedicine in India-the Apollo experience, Neurosurgery on the Web, 2001.
2. Bashshur RL, Armstrong PA, Youssef ZI. Telemedicine: Explorations in the use of telecommunications in health care. Charles C Thomas: Springfield, IL; 1975.
3. Bashshur R, Lovett J. Assessment of telemedicine: Results of the initial experience. *Aviation Space Environ Med* 1977;48:65–70.
4. Balas EA, Jaffery F, Pinciroli F. Patient care from a distance: Dasgupta A, et al.: Telemedicine 8 Indian Journal of Community Medicine Vol. 33, No. 1, January 2008 8 CMYK analysis of evidence. *Annu Meet Int Soc Technol Assess Health Care* 1996;12:17.
5. Mexrich RS, DeMarco JK, Negin S, et. al. Radiology on the information superhighway. *Radiology* 1995;195(1): 73–81.
6. Brown N. Telemedicine coming of age. TIE: September 28, 1996.

# 2

# PREDICTION OF HEART DISEASE

RAKSHI ANUJA DINESH, JAYASHREE SHANMUGAM, AND KUNAL BISWAS

## 2.1 Introduction

Numerous fields have profited from the rise of high-performance computing by discovering workable answers to their issues. This also applies to our system of healthcare. To help physicians make better diagnoses for therapeutic reasons, data-mining technologies have been created for the efficient examination of medical data (Kiruthika Devi et al., 2016). The use of data-mining techniques has been crucial in the study of cardiac disease. It is a commendable and excellent strategy in the research of heart-associated illness classification to identify any hidden medical information to look at the varied interpretations of healthy people and those with heart disease in the previously known medical data. The classification of heart disease provides a risky foundation for patient care. The two main methods used to predict the prevalence of heart disease based on the expression of medical data are statistics and machine learning. Healthcare research is expanding greatly to find the best solutions to lower mortality rates. Heart disease, which occurs from several causes, is one of the many illnesses that contribute significantly to the high mortality rates. The suggested approach tries to forecast cardiac disease more than previous techniques. Due to many subtle indications, heart disease treatments are now being delayed (Kalpana et al., 2021). The ability to forecast a patient's health state and take necessary action is supported by monitoring their health using data gathered from numerous resources. Predicting and diagnosing the illness is a problem in healthcare. Disease diagnosis is a complex undertaking that requires more precise findings. Therefore, its automation would be quite advantageous. This system's primary objective is to provide patients with a percentage-based prediction of their chances

DOI: 10.1201/9781032667508-2

of developing heart disease. This is accomplished using data-mining classification methods. The complete dataset is classified using two groups: yes and no. Through the use of machine learning classification algorithms, such as decision tree classification and Naive Bayes classification models, the classification approach is applied to the dataset. Utilising these models helps the categorisation technique's degree of accuracy rise. The categorisation and prediction techniques are both carried out by this model (Choudhary & Narayan Singh, 2020).

## 2.2 Risk Factors for Heart Disease

### 2.2.1 Controllable Risk Factors

*2.2.1.1 Smoking*   It has been studied and surveyed that smokers are two to four times more likely to have sudden heart attacks as compared to non-smokers. Smokers are more likely than non-smokers to die quickly after a heart attack, sometimes as quickly as one hour later. Compared to cigarette smokers, those who smoke pipes and cigars have a greater chance of dying from heart disease. Even if you don't smoke, exposure to environmental (or passive) tobacco smoke raises your chance of developing heart disease. Quit smoking to lower your chance of developing heart disease (*Heart Disease Risk Factors*, n.d.).

*2.2.1.2 High Blood Pressure*   The heart experiences increased effort or stress from high blood pressure, which over time, causes the organ to become bigger and weaker. High blood pressure sufferers also have a higher risk of stroke, heart attack, renal failure, and congestive heart failure. The risk of heart attack or stroke is multiplied when obesity, smoking, high blood cholesterol, and/or diabetes are present. Learning to control high blood pressure by making lifestyle adjustments, managing stress, or using medication is recommended (*Heart Disease Risk Factors*, n.d.).

*2.2.1.3 Stress*   Heart disease may be exacerbated by stress. Everyone encounters stress and is a necessary component of being a person, of living, and of engaging with the outside world. Our stress response has an impact on our health, particularly the risk of heart disease. It is advisable that every individual must control and regulate their everyday stress level to avoid chronic stress, which may be detrimental to the cardiac health system (*Heart Disease Risk Factors,* n.d).

*2.2.1.4 Obesity and Overweight*   Even without any other risk factors, those with extra body fat—especially around the waist—are more likely to develop heart disease. Weight gain makes the heart work harder and causes blood pressure to rise. As weight grows, blood cholesterol and triglyceride levels rise as well, lowering the "good" cholesterol. Additionally, diabetes is more prone to develop in overweight individuals. Patients may improve their health and lower their risk for heart disease by losing only 10 to 20 pounds (*Heart Disease Risk Factors*, n.d.). In obese patients, it is advisable to alter their diet by including nutritional food items, adopt a lower-fat diet, get regular exercise, and further consult a practitioner in case of weight issues.

*2.2.1.5 High Blood Sugar*   Diabetes significantly raises the risk for heart disease and stroke and is a complicating factor for heart disease. Numerous Americans live with diabetes but are unaware of it. Your risk for heart disease may be decreased via changes to your lifestyle and medical treatment of diabetes. Speak with your doctor if you haven't had a diabetic screening yet (*Heart Disease Risk Factors*, n.d.). In case there is a diabetes history in your family, it is recommended to test sugar levels sooner, as there is a high chance of having high blood sugar if it exists in your family line. If you do have diabetes, educate yourself as much as you can on how to control it. There are a lot of options for managing diabetes and lowering the risk of heart disease.

### *2.2.2 Uncontrollable Risk Factors*

*2.2.2.1 Age*   Older persons have a higher risk of cardiovascular disease (CVD) due to the decline of cardiovascular function brought on by aging (Curtis et al., 2018; North & Sinclair, 2012). Along with atherosclerosis, stroke, and myocardial infarction, the prevalence of CVD has also been demonstrated to rise with aging in both men and women (Yazdanyar & Newman, 2009). Arteries and the heart might change as we age. For instance, as you age, your heart can no longer beat as quickly as it could when you were younger during physical exertion or stressful situations. However, normal aging has little effect on the heart rate (the average number of beats per minute) during rest. A person's risk of heart disease may rise with aging-related changes. The accumulation of fatty deposits in artery walls over a long period is one of the main causes of heart disease. Arteriosclerosis, also known as artery hardening, or increasing stiffness of the major arteries, is the most typical change due to aging. As we age, hypertension, or high blood pressure, becomes increasingly typical.

*2.2.2.2 Gender*   CVD is one of the main causes of mortality around the world. Women typically have a lower incidence of CVD than males, however, following acute cardiovascular events, women have greater mortality and poorer prognosis. Different CVDs, such as coronary heart disease (CHD), stroke, heart failure, and aortic illnesses, exhibit these gender variances. Gender consideration is crucial for the prevention, diagnosis, treatment, and management of CVD since these gender disparities have raised significant concerns (Gao et al., 2019). Men are more likely than women to have a heart attack, and they do so earlier in life. After menopause, the mortality rate from cardiac disease among women rises, although it still lags behind that of males.

### *2.2.3 Additional Cautions*

Regular or heavy drinking of **alcohol** may increase blood pressure, bring on heart failure, and result in a stroke. Additionally, it supports obesity, alcoholism, accidents, and suicide. It is recommended that drinking is safer in moderate amounts (no more than two drinks for men and one drink for women on a daily basis). One drink is defined as 12 ounces of beer, 1 ounce of 100-proof alcohol, or 1 ounce of 80-proof alcohol. Early **birth control pill** formulations that had greater progesterone and oestrogen dosages raised the risk of heart disease and stroke, especially in women who smoked regularly (*Drinking Too Much Alcohol Can Harm Your Health. Learn the Facts | CDC*, n.d.). Unless women who use them also smoke or have high blood pressure,

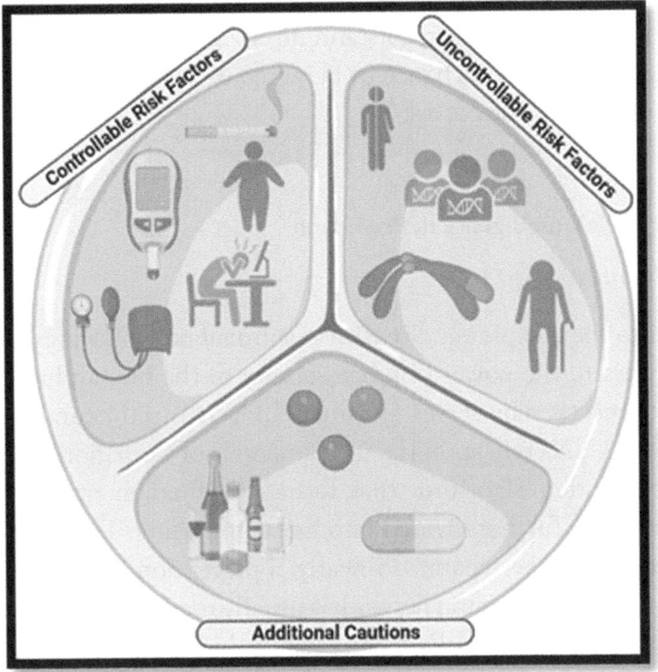


**Figure 2.1** Risk factors for heart disease. (Illustration by the author.)

the risk of using more recent oral contraceptives is much reduced. It is advisable that women should check their triglyceride level, blood pressure level, and glucose levels annually if on birth control pills and also smoking. It is recommended to give up smoking if you use birth control pills and smoke to lower your chance of developing heart disease. After menopause, when oestrogen production naturally declines, it has been shown that **sex hormones** have a role in the development of heart disease in women (*Heart Disease Risk Factors*, n.d.). The risk factors for heart disease are shown in Figure 2.1.

## 2.3 Materials and Methods or Research Work

To start the task, a variety of data has been gathered in every area related to the system's objective. Major causes and effects in resulting heart health are the first focus of the present study. Some of the unavoidable causes and variables of heart health are dependent upon age, sex, and family history. On the other hand, some of the dependent variables that could be controlled and are equally responsible for heart-related ailments and diseases are heart rate and blood pressure, which has a chance of being controlled per specific guidelines and medical protocols.

## 2.4 Artificial Intelligence in Prediction

### 2.4.1 Neural Network

Owing to the complex and sensitive neuronal networks present in the human brain, the power of processability of the human brain is significant and thereby serves as a model for artificial neural networks (ANNs). ANNs rely upon the fundamentals of formation of a single-layer perception algorithm that forms the fundamental processing unit, which is further divided into linear segments. To tackle certain issues that can't be separated linearly, a perception model Multilayer Perception (MLP) neural network is usually used. Some of the aspects encompassed in the MLPs are the inputs, hidden and the output layers, respectively (Kalpana et al., 2021).

*2.4.1.1 Convolution Neural Network*    It is appropriate to refer to the task of predicting a patient's CHD as a binary classification task. In the context of supervised learning, the neural network has demonstrated effectiveness as a classifier in specific circumstances (Hinton et al., 2015). Recent studies showed that neural networks with application-specific settings, such as many hidden layers, have significantly improved in several domains. Image processing, audio processing, and time series prediction are applications of neural networks that have had substantial success. Various deep-learning architectures have undergone thorough training and fine-tuning using relatively larger datasets.

The transfer of input data via hidden layers and assessment of error at the output layer make up how an ANN functions (He et al., 2016; Iandola, 2016; Szegedy et al., 2017). The backpropagated error by the output layer is then used by a gradient descent method for an iterative update of the layer weights. Numerous experiments and analyses have suggested numerous adjustments to the gradient descent technique, including a decrease in overfitting, timing the training procedure, making the layers non-linear, seeing the hidden layers, and other changes.

The operation of deep neural networks is still poorly understood, despite the apparent success of its applications. Additionally, it is discovered that the training networks are easily overfitted as a result of the deep architecture's millions of parameters. When the examples are insufficient, the issue worsens. To address this problem, numerous algorithms have been developed. One of the often utilised methods is data augmentation which artificially populates new tiny datasets based on the examples already there (Krizhevsky et al., 2017; Radford et al., 2015). However, when we are explicitly discussing a biological application like clinical datasets, such techniques are not believable even though this technique produces substantially superior instances. The increased measurements of a CHD phenotype, such as platelet count, might not match the patient's probable range of readings, for example. The basic distinction between the principles behind platelet-count readings and statistical generation is what led to this predicament. Small or distorted datasets result in subpar training, which in turn produces subpar and erroneous categorisation. Compared to other applications like semantic labeling, picture synthesis, etc., a false prediction in medical research carries a substantially larger penalty.

### 2.4.2 Bayesian Classifiers

Data mining is a method of knowledge discovery used to examine data and turn it into usable information. Given a patient dataset, the present study aims to estimate the likelihood of developing the cardiac disease (Jabbar et al., 2011). In practice, data mining's main objectives are predictions and descriptions (Srinivas et al., 2011). Data-mining prediction uses variables or characteristics in the dataset to identify unknowable or potential values for other properties (Vijiyarani et al., 2013). The focus of the description is on finding patterns that explain the data so that people can comprehend it. From historical data on individuals with heart disease, the system can extract the hidden information associated with diseases using Bayesian classifiers. The class membership probabilities are predicted by Bayesian classifiers in a manner that statistically determines the likelihood that a given sample belongs to a certain class. The Bayes theorem may be used to calculate the likelihood that a suggested diagnosis is accurate given an observation. The Naive Bayes classifier, a straightforward probabilistic, is used to classify data using Bayes' theorem as a foundation. The existence of any other feature is determined using a naive Bayesian classifier. The main Naive Bayes classifier approach is appropriate when a higher level of input dimension and a more effective outcome are desired (Liu et al., 2016; Maheswari & Pitchai, 2018; Pattekari & Parveen, 2012). The Naive Bayes model recognises the physical traits and attributes of heart disease patients. It provides the potential characteristic for the anticipated state for each input. The application of the Naive Bayes algorithm on patient data is shown in Figure 2.2.

### 2.4.3 Decision Tree

With great success, researchers have seen the treatment of heart diseases with the presentation of the decision tree approach (Shouman et al., 2010). The tree-like structure of a typical decision tree comprises an internal node, a leaf node, and a branch, respectively. It is understood that each leaf node denotes the predicted aspect of classes

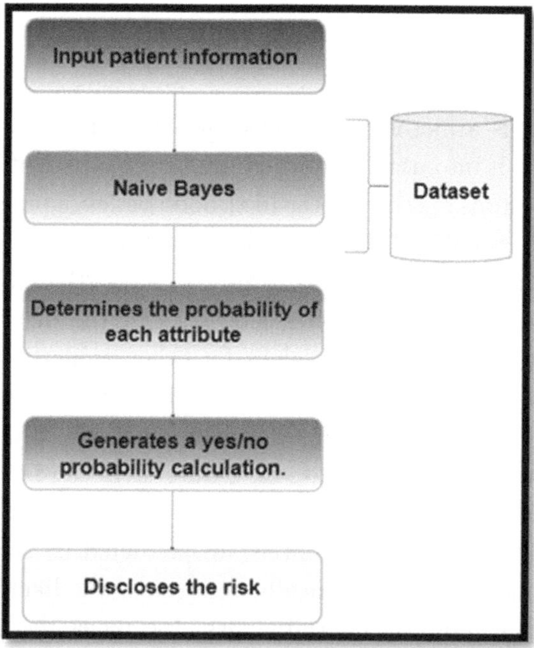


**Figure 2.2**    Naive Bayes method application to patient data. (Illustration by the author.)

or class distributions. On the other hand, each internal node denotes a test on an attribute that is utilised for applications, whereas each branch nodes denotes an attribute value. It is further understood that the categorisation proceeds towards the tree relying on the predictive attribute value, when initiated at the root node. Some of the aspects which enable the trimming of the decision trees encompasses data categorisation, decision tree category selection, data partitioning, and request for the reduction of fault trimming aspects.

There are two types of classification techniques: supervised and unsupervised methods. Chi merge and entropy are used in supervised classification techniques, while similar width and identical frequency are used in unsupervised approaches. Testing is done throughout the data partitioning with or without voting. Gini Index, Information Improvement, and Gain Ratio are three kinds of decision trees that are put to the test. To give more closed decision rules, less error cutting is helpful. The implementation of the ID3 algorithm on patient data is shown in Figure 2.3.

### 2.4.4 Support Vector Machine

Recently, support vector machines (SVMs) have drawn a lot of interest (Cristianini & Shawe-Taylor, 2000; Vapnik, 1999; Iyer et al., 2015; Majali et al., 2015) due to their success in a range of pattern categorisation tasks. With considerable success, they have been used to solve a variety of issues, including hand-written character recognition, bioinformatics, and automated voice recognition. The SVM algorithm is a supervised machine learning method that classifies information best by generating the margin between two data clusters and predicts the occurrence of heart disease by mapping the disease-predicting features on a multidimensional hyperplane. This technique uses nonlinear functions referred to as kernels to achieve great precision.

### 2.4.5 Hybrid

One of the biggest problems in the healthcare sector is the prediction of heart disease (Alzahani et al., 2014; Liu et al., 2016; Swathi, 2015). Researchers are employing various data-mining approaches to diagnose heart disease as a result of the rising mortality of heart disease

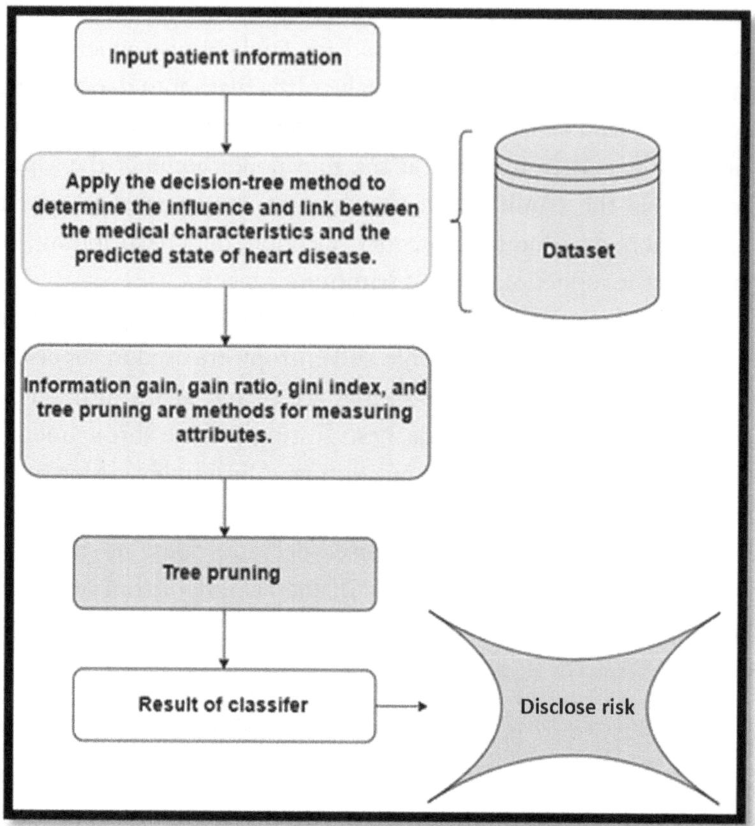


**Figure 2.3**    ID3 algorithm implementation concerning patient data. (Illustration by the author.)

patients around the globe. Each method has advantages and disadvantages of its own. There are certain functions built into each algorithm utilised by each approach that are useful for diagnosing heart disease. The results of each algorithm are pooled and evaluated for the most accurate analysis of heart disease. In this context, combining the output is referred to as "hybridisation." Heart disease diagnostics using hybrid data-mining approaches may provide encouraging results.

## 2.5 Conclusion

Owing to the effectiveness and precision of the MLP model, machine learning algorithms have seen great improvements in technological interventions, which has been discussed in the chapter. Also, it has been studied that algorithms enable the effective output of the corresponding input value performed by the consumer, which is trustworthy and reliable in nature. The frequency of the utilisation of the system—the more the utilisation of the system, the better the individual would be aware about the heart health status—results in the minimisation of mortality rate due to heart health aspects. One of the algorithmic approaches studied in the present chapter is Naive Bayes classifier and decision tree classification, which were shown to aid in the prediction of the likelihood of a patient having heart disease. In the nutshell, the utilisation of the different merged methods in the single algorithm resulted into the production of more accurate and robust data output, which could play a role in predicting and thereby minimising sudden heart attacks and ailments. This chapter plays a critical role in designing a roadmap for a therapeutic regime in heart-health diagnostics and effective treatments in days to come.

## Acknowledgements

Authors thank Department of Biotechnology, Sathyabama Institute of Science and Technology, Chennai and International Research Centre, Centre for Nanoscience and Nanotechnology, Sathyabama Institute of Science and Technology, Chennai for carrying out the work.

## Conflict of Interest

Authors declare that there are no conflict of interest(s) of any kind between the authors.

# References

Alzahani, S. M., Althopity, A., Alghamdi, A., Alshehri, B., & Aljuaid, S. (2014). An overview of data mining techniques applied for heart disease diagnosis and prediction. *Lecture Notes on Information Theory, 2(4)*, 310–315.

Choudhary, G., & Narayan Singh, S. (2020). Prediction of heart disease using machine learning algorithms. *Proceedings of the International Conference on Smart Technologies in Computing, Electrical and Electronics, ICSTCEE 2020*, 197–202. https://doi.org/10.1109/ICSTCEE49637.2020.9276802

Cristianini, N., & Shawe-Taylor, J. (2000). *An introduction to support vector machines and other kernel-based learning methods*. Cambridge university press.

Curtis, A. B., Karki, R., Hattoum, A., & Sharma, U. C. (2018). Arrhythmias in patients ≥ 80 years of age: pathophysiology, management, and outcomes. *Journal of the American College of Cardiology, 71*(*18*), 2041–2057.

*Drinking too much alcohol can harm your health. Learn the facts | CDC*. (n.d.). https://www.cdc.gov/alcohol/fact-sheets/alcohol-use.htm

Gao, Z., Chen, Z., Sun, A., & Deng, X. (2019). Gender differences in cardiovascular disease. *Medicine in Novel Technology and Devices, 4*, 100025. https://doi.org/10.1016/j.medntd.2019.100025

He, K., Zhang, X., Ren, S., & Sun, J. (2016). Deep residual learning for image recognition. *Proceedings of the IEEE Conference on Computer Vision and Pattern Recognition*, 770–778.

*Heart Disease Risk Factors*. (n.d.). https://www.mclaren.org/main/heart-disease-risk-factors

Hinton, G., LeCun, Y., & Bengio, Y. (2015). Deep learning. *Nature, 521*(*7553*), 436–444.

Iandola, F. (2016). *Exploring the design space of deep convolutional neural networks at large scale*. University of California, Berkeley.

Iyer, A., Jeyalatha, S., & Sumbaly, R. (2015). Diagnosis of diabetes using classification mining techniques. *ArXiv Preprint ArXiv:1502.03774*.

Jabbar, M. A., Chandra, P., & Deekshatulu, B. L. (2011). Cluster based association rule mining for heart attack prediction. *Journal of Theoretical and Applied Information Technology, 32*(*2*), 196–201.

Kalpana, P., Shiyam Vignesh, S., Surya, L. M. P., & Vishnu Prasad, V. (2021). Retraction: prediction of heart disease using machine learning. *Journal of Physics: Conference Series, 1916*(1), 1275–1278. https://doi.org/10.1088/1742-6596/1916/1/012022

Kiruthika Devi, S., Krishnapriya, S., & Kalita, D. (2016). Prediction of heart disease using data mining techniques. *Indian Journal of Science and Technology, 9*(39). https://doi.org/10.17485/ijst/2016/v9i39/102078

Krizhevsky, A., Sutskever, I., & Hinton, G. E. (2017). Imagenet classification with deep convolutional neural networks. *Communications of the ACM, 60*(*6*), 84–90.

Liu, X., Lu, R., Ma, J., Chen, L., & Qin, B. (2016). Privacy-preserving patient-centric clinical decision support system on Naïve Bayesian classification. *IEEE Journal of Biomedical and Health Informatics, 20*(2), 655–668. https://doi.org/10.1109/JBHI.2015.2407157

Maheswari, S., & Pitchai, R. (2018). Heart disease prediction system using decision tree and Naive Bayes algorithm. *Current Medical Imaging Formerly Current Medical Imaging Reviews, 15*(8), 712–717. https://doi.org/10.2174/1573405614666180322141259

Majali, J., Niranjan, R., Phatak, V., & Tadakhe, O. (2015). Data mining techniques for diagnosis and prognosis of cancer. *International Journal of Advanced Research in Computer and Communication Engineering, 4*(3), 613–615. https://doi.org/10.17148/ijarcce.2015.43147

North, B. J., & Sinclair, D. A. (2012). The intersection between aging and cardiovascular disease. *Circulation Research, 110*(*8*), 1097–1108.

Pattekari, S. A., & Parveen, A. (2012). Prediction system for heart disease using Naïve Bayes. *International Journal of Advanced Computer and Mathematical Sciences, 3(3)*, 290–294.

Radford, A., Metz, L., & Chintala, S. (2015). Unsupervised representation learning with deep convolutional generative adversarial networks. *ArXiv Preprint ArXiv:1511.06434*.

Shouman, M., Turner, T., & Stocker, R. (2010). Using decision tree for diagnosing heart disease patients. *Conferences in Research and Practice in Information Technology Series, 121*, 23–30.

Srinivas, K., Rao, G. R., & Govardhan, A. (2011). Survey on prediction of heart morbidity using data mining techniques. *International Journal of Data Mining & Knowledge Management Process (IJDKP), 1(3)*, 14–34.

Swathi, D., Yogish, & Sreeraj. (2015). *Predictive Data Mining Procedures for the Prediction of Coronary Artery Disease.*

Szegedy, C., Ioffe, S., Vanhoucke, V., & Alemi, A. A. (2017). Inception-v4, inception-resnet and the impact of residual connections on learning. *Thirty-First AAAI Conference on Artificial Intelligence.*

Vapnik, V. (1999). *The nature of statistical learning theory.* Springer science & business media.

Vijiyarani, S., & Sudha, S., & Research Scholar, M. P. (2013). Disease prediction in data mining technique – A survey. *International Journal of Computer Applications & Information Technology, II(I)*, 2278–7720.

Yazdanyar, A., & Newman, A. B. (2009). The burden of cardiovascular disease in the elderly: morbidity, mortality, and costs. *Clinics in Geriatric Medicine, 25(4)*, 563–577.

# 3

# DETECTING DRUG-ARTEMISININ RESISTANCE BASED ON THE DNA BARCODE SEQUENCE OF PLASMODIUM FALCIPARUM USING A MACHINE LEARNING ALGORITHM

LAILIL MUFLIKHAH

## 3.1 Introduction

*Plasmodium falciparum* is a parasitic viral infection for malaria. This type of disease exists in countries with tropical climates, including Indonesia. Various efforts have been made to reduce the number of deaths from this disease with intensive treatment. One of the causes of the high case rate is the *Plasmodium* parasite's resistance to anti-malarial drugs. These types of anti-malarial drugs are classified as antibiotics, and an appropriate regulation is needed including information regarding the large number of genetic variants of this parasite that hinders the development of effective malaria vaccines. The antigenic variation in this parasite significantly hinders vaccine research—many alleles effectively evade vaccine-induced allele-specific immunity. *P. falciparum* is a potential antigen candidate for vaccine development [1]. Resistance of *P. falciparum* to anti-malarial drugs is one of the causes of the high mortality rate in endemic areas. One of the main causes is a mutation in the gene of the parasite so that the performance is not effective in the target region. Several studies related to drug resistance were carried out *in vivo*, *in vitro*, and *in silico* using the bioinformatics method to find the characteristics of these parasites. Molecular biology research was carried out in the wet lab to determine the level of polymorphism of the anti-malarial treatment target genes [2, 3]. Furthermore, based on a sufficiently



DOI: 10.1201/9781032667508-3

high-volume dataset, research using a computational approach was conducted, starting from image data (haploid), clinical data, and chemical data analysis to DNA sequence data (genetic variants) using machine learning (ML) algorithms [1, 4–8]. Therefore, we proposed to research the study of genetic variant analysis against *Plasmodium* parasite resistance in target genes and anti-malarial drug artemisinin with a computational approach using ML algorithms.

This chapter is organized as follows. The research background is presented in the first section of this paper. Then, problem formulation is the research question for this study with material and research methods provided. The material consists of the theory of anti-malarial drugs, DNA barcoding, and ML algorithms. Finally, we provide a solution, evaluation of results, and a conclusion.

### 3.2 Problem Formulation

The limitation of anti-malarial drugs is resistance to *Plasmodium*, which is caused by mutations in the target gene. By identifying the uniqueness of the DNA sequence, DNA barcoding is used to look for motifs to determine the relationship among the mutations and drug resistance. Therefore, the problems of this research include how to model for the detection of anti-malarial drug resistance based on DNA barcodes with a high level of performance using representative ML algorithms such as K-Nearest Neighbor (KNN), Naïve Bayes, Support Vector Machine (SVM), decision tree C4.5 and Random Forest (RF).

### 3.3 Anti-Malarial Drug

Treatment of malaria through drug therapy aims to eliminate the *Plasmodium* parasite in the host. However, resistance of the *P. falciparum* to anti-folate resulted in the sequential acquisition of mutations in the target gene [1]. The high mutation rate of this type of *Plasmodium* parasite species causes resistance, so a combination of anti-malarial drugs is carried out. With the possibility of the immunity of malaria parasites to anti-malarial drugs, The World Health Organization (WHO) has advised the use of an approved combination of artemisinin, Artemisinin Combination Therapy (ACT).

The efficacies of many anti-malarial drugs are limited by drug resistance, and recent evidence suggests that parasites are becoming resistant to the newest agents. However, the extent of resistance varies, such that in many cases, drugs with resistance concerns offer effective treatment and control of malaria. Resistance has been described for nearly all available drugs and is discussed later in the chapter. For many drugs, the extent of resistance is uncertain and mechanisms of resistance are unknown, and, thus, the opportunity to glean data from the ten International Centers of Excellence for Malaria Research (ICEMR) surveillance sites is highly valuable. Resistance can be assessed by clinical trials comparing anti-malarial efficacies of different agents, *ex vivo/in vitro* assessment of sensitivities of cultured *P. falciparum*, evaluation of genetic polymorphisms associated with resistance, or by assessing the selective pressure of anti-malarial treatment on subsequent infections. Studies considering all these factors have shed light on the extent of resistance and mechanisms of resistance [2].

## 3.4 DNA Barcode

Each organism has the same DNA sequence. Unification of the DNA sequence can identify the organism. DNA barcoding is a strategy to recognize and give auto-validation for living beings. It has a specific region, and the length of the sequence is between 300 and 400 bps (branch point sequence). The barcoding-based protein measurement method achieve ultrasensitive detection down to the single molecule level by converting protein signals into barcoded oligo probes and amplifying the signals with nucleic acid amplification. Low-abundance surface markers of cancer cells or rare tumor cells can be detected using this method [3]. The Weissleder group developed photo-cleavable DNA-barcoded antibodies that are specifically capable of recognizing multi-plexed cell biomarkers. After that, DNA has been cleaved by light (less than 365 nm) and released into solution; gel electrophoresis can be used to analyze it. They also came up with an amplification-free method to profile more than 90 proteins in single cells using DNA-barcoded antibodies and NanoString's fluorescent readout to study the drug response pathway and inter- and intra-tumor heterogeneity in clinical samples [4].

## 3.5 Machine Learning

ML is a field in artificial intelligence, which is the science and technique of making machines think like humans. ML focuses on the automated acquisition of knowledge. ML does not only discuss how the methods in ML work, but in applying these methods, ML always intersects with other fields such as statistics, economics, biology, and others [5].

The ML algorithm is based on the input provided. In the method, there are two approaches, namely supervised and unsupervised learning. The difference between the two approaches is the type of learning being carried out. For example: training data: $(x_1, y_1)$, $(x_n, y_n)$, $x_i \varepsilon R_d$, and $y_i$ is a label [9]. A computer program teaches the machine to learn through the generated data, for description or prediction tasks. Unsupervised learning is an ML technique that does not require user supervision of the model, allowing it to work alone to discover previously undetected patterns and information. Unsupervised learning is primarily concerned with unlabeled data. Supervised learning is an ML technique that learns from labelled training data to assist users in predicting outcomes for unexpected data. In supervised learning, the machine is trained using properly "labelled" data that are tagged with the correct answer or prediction result. Supervised learning can be thought of as learning in the presence of a supervisor or teacher who always directs the correct answer, as illustrated in Figure 3.1 [4]. This study implemented the representative supervised learning method including KNN, Naïve Bayes, SVM, decision tree C4.5., and RF.

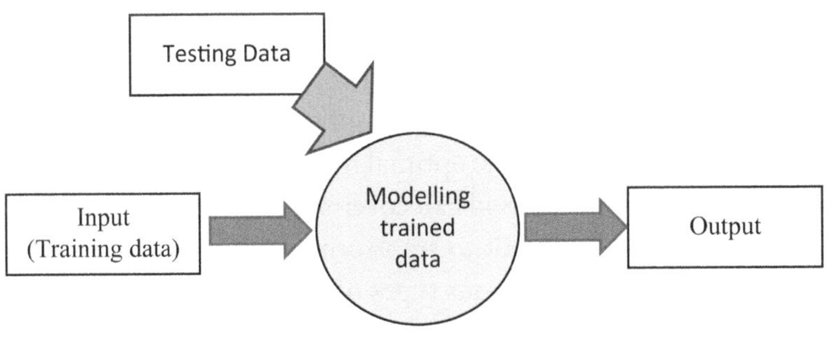


**Figure 3.1**   Illustration of a supervised learning method [4].

### 3.5.1 K-Nearest Neighbor

The KNN classifier is a supervised learning algorithm that is based on a comparison of the characteristics of objects that are divided into their categories to predict the label or category of the new information object. This method of classification is considered lazy because the construction for modeling retrieved from training data is not necessary. The majority of the training data object class in the KNN data determines the class value of the new data [10, 11].

### 3.5.2 Naïve Bayes Classifier

Naïve Bayes is a supervised learning method that can classify data. The method uses unconditional and conditional probability to construct the classifier model. The principal concept is the independence of each event (unconditional probability) with a very strong (naïve) hypothesis [12]. The model is constructed based on Eq. 3.1.

$$P(C|X) = \frac{P(C)P(X|C)}{P(X)} \tag{3.1}$$

where $X$ is attributed, and $C$ is class.

The posterior probability value of each class is maximized in the Bayes classifier. It is defined in the formula in the Eq. 3.2.

$$H_{MAP} = \arg\max P(C|x_1, x_2, \ldots x_n) \arg\max \text{Pnaïve} \prod_{i=1}^{n} P(x_i|C) \tag{3.2}$$

### 3.5.3 Support Vector Machine

Another supervised learning method for classification is the SVM classifier [13]. Initially, the function splits the input space into two classes. This method seeks the optimal hyperplane function. The function developed in this method can cover non-linear classification. The kernel trick function is built to transform a sufficiently high dimension into a vector space. Various types of kernel functions can be used with the SVM classifier—in this study, the Radial Basis Function (RBF) kernel function is used.

In the SVM classifier, each class is labelled y-naïve e {−1, +1} for naïve = 1, 2, n, where n is total data. The label is divided from the hyperplane (support vector), as defined in Eq. 3.4 and Eq. 3.5.

$$w.x + b = 0 \tag{3.3}$$

The data point $x_i$ is set to −1, as shown in Eq. (3.4):

$$w.x_i + b \leq -1 \tag{3.4}$$

The data point $x_i$ is set to +1, as shown in Eq. (3.5):

$$w.x_i + b \geq +1 \tag{3.5}$$

The maximum margin is considered the maximum distance of the hyperplane to close the data object.

$$\frac{1}{\| w \|} \tag{3.6}$$

The basic intention of the SVM classifier is to transform the data $x$ into the high-dimensional vector space function $< D\,(x_i)$. Thus, the new vector space data are represented in the objective function. Training the data is the process of learning to search for support vectors in the form of a hyperplane by means of a dot product among the data of a new vector space using a kernel function as defined in the formula (Eq. 3.7).

$$K\left(x_i.x_j\right) = \Phi\left(x_i\right).\Phi\left(x_j\right) \tag{3.7}$$

The RBF is a kernel trick used as shown in Eq. 3.8.

$$K\left(X_i \cdot X_j\right) = \exp\left(-\left(\frac{\|X_i - X_j\|^2}{2\sigma^2}\right)\right) \tag{3.8}$$

The next step is to apply a sequential SVM algorithm to build predictions such as the Hessian matrix, the iteration to get the maximum of the minimum error rates, or the maximum, $(|\,5a\,|) <e$ and then compute the test and training data to get the bias and similarity between these datasets. A set of classes is obtained [14–17].

### 3.5.4 Decision Tree C4.5

C5.0 is a decision tree classifier method that goes beyond C4.5 and is built in the recursive division of a structured tree. This method uses 'divide and conquer' in its principal concept to provide features such as a node into smaller subsets in the same classes. The data are then split to the branch that determines the chosen decision. The tree is completed by leaf nodes as a decision termination, which is used to determine the outcome after a set of decisions. The C5.0 decision tree classifier model is an extended C4.5 decision tree algorithm, as proposed by Quinlan in 1993 [18]. It implemented methods for boosting and narrowing as well as the asymmetric costs for specific errors [19].

### 3.5.5 Random Forest

Random Forest (RF) is a collection of tree predictors with a uniform distribution in one forest. This tree is constructed without pruning of the classification and regression trees (CART) decision tree. The RF is a supervised learning method for evaluating the performance of feature selection in hepatoma detection. One of the strengths of RF is its robustness [20] and predictability [21]. The RF method is built from several decision trees by selecting the number of F features randomly. This means that not all features are used to build the tree. The value of F affects the performance of the RF. If the F value is too small (F $\ll$ M attribute), the correlation value from the tree will tend to be a small value (small correlation). Otherwise, if the F value is too large (F $\gg$ M attribute), the correlation value from the tree will tend to be a great value (strong correlation) [22]. Furthermore, the F value and the number of all attributes, M, can be determined by Eq. 3.9.

$$F = \log_2\left(/M + 1\right) \tag{3.9}$$

### 3.6 Problem Solution

In general, this research uses ML algorithms. Conceptually, this study began by collecting sequence data from DNA barcode for artemisinin at MalariaGEN sites. The data were generated to construct a classifier model (representative ML algorithms) for detection. Then, we evaluated the performance through measuring accuracy, precision, recall, and f1-score.

**Table 3.1**   DNA Barcode Sequences Data of Artemisinin Drug

| STATE | SPECIES | GEN BARCODE | STATUS |
|---|---|---|---|
| RCN03189 | Pf | AAXXXXXATXAACGCGXATXAGGAGCGGCCAACCTCATTXCACXCATGCAA | Resistant |
| RCN03192 | Pf | AGGTGGGXCTAAGTAACGTAACXCXGXCTCXCAXTAXXCXXXCAACXAAT | Sensitive |
| RCN00121 | Pf | GGXXGACXXXAGTGTGXGAXTGTGACACTCAATCATATTXATTXTXTAXXA | Sensitive |
| RCN00122 | Pf | XAGTGGGXXTXXGXAXCAXCXGXAXGXCXCXXAXTGXXXCTXXXXTGAAT | Sensitive |
| RCN00123 | Pf | GGXCANTGTXAANCNGCNTNATTNGCXCCCTNTCATGTCGCNTTNGNGCAX | Sensitive |
| RCN00124 | Pf | AAXNNNGXACXNACGCNNAAXGXAGAGTCAGNGACNATCTCGCTACNXNT | Sensitive |

### 3.6.1 Dataset

This research was conducted to detect the anti-malarial drug resistance (artemisinin) against *P. falciparum* using ML algorithms. The dataset used for this study is taken from the MalariaNET database including 3176 resistant and 3787 sensitive data. As an illustration, the DNA barcode sequences are shown in Table 3.1. The length of sequences is about 100 bps and consist of Adenine (A), Thimine (T), Guanine (G), Cytosine (C), and another character (X).

### 3.6.2 Classifier Model for Detection

The model was constructed from generated sequence data based on the method. In the KNN algorithm, the class is detemined based on similarity using a distance matrix. Using decision tree C4.5, the node is selected from the entropy calculation. The higher level of the node in tree, the higher the entropy value. Another ML is SVM, which builds a classifier model based on the hyperplane function to define label class. Furthermore, the RF is an ensemble method under the decisision tree collection. As a visual, the representative model is plotted in two-dimensional graphics as shown in Figure 3.2, Figure 3.3, Figure 3.4, and Figure 3.5.

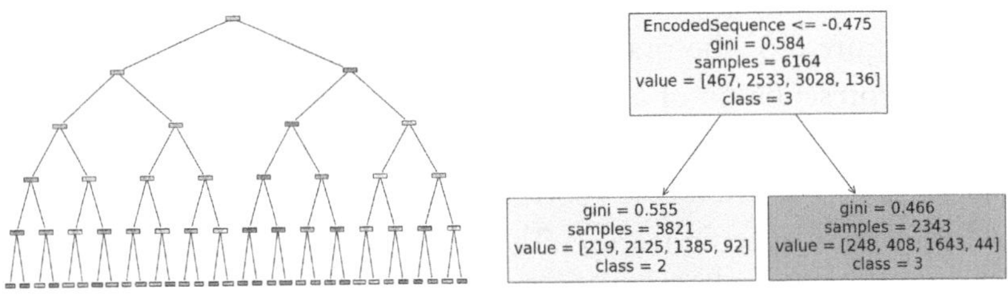


**Figure 3.2**   Decision tree C4.5. Classifier of (a) the result model and (b) the structure model.

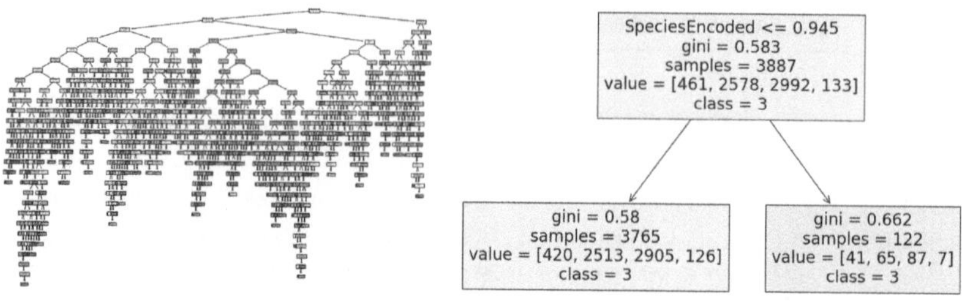

**Figure 3.3**   Random forest classifier of (a) the result model and (b) the structure model.

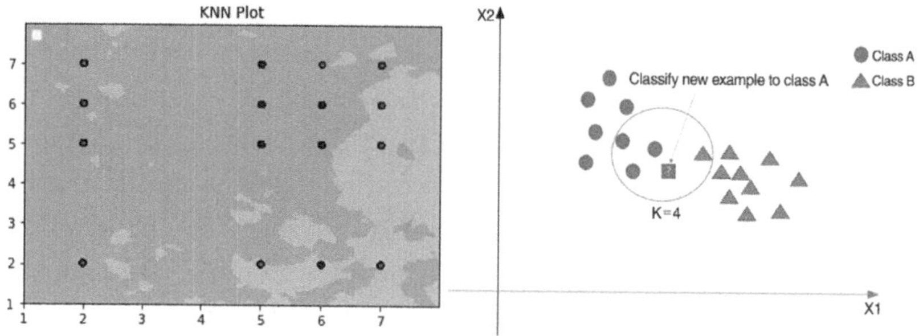

**Figure 3.4**   KNN classifier of (a) the result model and (b) the structure model.

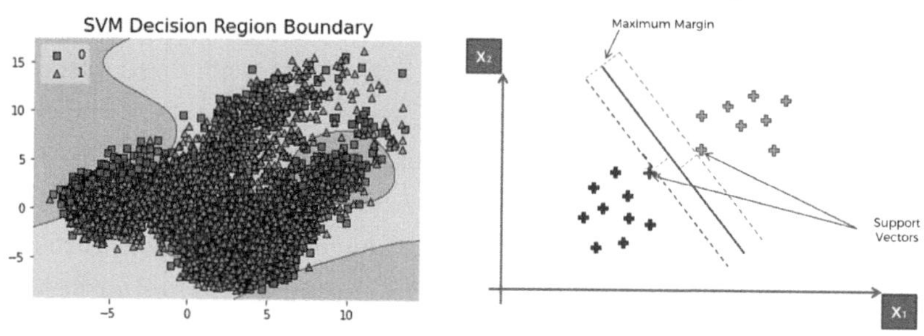

**Figure 3.5**   SVM classifier of (a) the result model and (b) the structure model.

In Figure 3.3, the graphic result of a decision tree classifier is a visual representation of a tree-like structure. Several elements inside the graphical representation include root nodes, internal nodes, leaf nodes, and branches. The root node of the tree represents the first decision on a specific feature. Then, the internal node has branches associated with splitting criteria greater than a certain threshold. Finally, the leaf node is the final predicted class. Figure 3.2a is a model of decision tree C.4.5, and (b) is a grammatically structured model of the C4.5. classifier.

The RF classifier is an aggregated decision tree for prediction. The graphical result of an RF classifier, as shown in Figure 3.3a, consists of a collection of decision tree diagrams, each representing an ensemble in one of trees as shown in Figure 3.3b. This method builds prediction by combining the results from individual trees using majority voting in this study.

Visualization of the KNN classifier is shown in Figure 3.4(a), and an illustration of how the method works in classification based on their proximity in the feature space and the decision boundaries in data distribution are shown in Figure 3.4b. Each point represents data, and the position is related to its feature values. Different classes are shown below that illustrate regions closest to each data point.

The graphic result of an SVM classifier for the drug resistance prediction is shown in Figure 3.5a and the illustration of how the SVM work is performed by the hyperplane as a decision boundary in Figure 3.5b. The dataset is displayed in a scatter plot and the feature values are represented to their position. A hyperplane separates the different binary classes in the feature space. Support vectors are the data points that are crucial to determine the position of the decision boundary from a class. Its role is defining the margin.

### 3.6.3 *Evaluation of Result*

One of the evaluation methods required in data composition is a $k$-fold cross-validation. The testing data used as $m$ folds and the training data used as $k$ folds. The data are divided by $k$ parts and are then iterated, for $k$ iterations, in the different folds. In this study, the total number of folds were divided into two, one being training data and the other being testing data [23].

To know the performance of the classification method, we need to evaluate the results. The evaluation is employed by comparing the predicted results with the actual label (ground truth) [24] as shown in Figure 3.6. The evaluation method will produce a scalar value or curve. The evaluation method is useful for interpreting training results or comparing classification algorithms.

<table>
<tr><td rowspan="3"></td><td></td><td colspan="2">Prediction</td></tr>
<tr><td></td><td>Positive</td><td>Negative</td></tr>
<tr><td></td></tr>
</table>

| | | Prediction | |
| --- | --- | --- | --- |
| | | **Positive** | **Negative** |
| **Ground Truth** | **Positive** | TP | FN |
| | **Negative** | FP | TN |

**Figure 3.6**  Confusion matrix.

The comparison between prediction results and ground truth in binary classification can be divided into four categories:

1. True Positive (TP): If the predicted class is positive and the ground truth is positive, then it is a True value.
2. False Negative (FN): If the predicted class is negative and the ground truth is positive, then it is an Error–Type 2.
3. False Positive (FP): If the predicted class is positive and the ground truth is negative, then it is an Error–Type 1.
4. True Negative (TN): If the predicted class is negative and the ground truth is negative, then it is a True value.

Then, the performance measurement on this research was used, including accuracy, precision, recall, and f1-score as stated in Eq. 3.10, Eq. 3.11, Eq. 3.12, and Eq. 3.13 [24].

$$Accuracy = \frac{TP + TN}{TP + TN + FP + FN} \qquad \text{Eq. (3.10)}$$

$$Precision = \frac{TP}{TP + FN} \qquad \text{Eq. (3.11)}$$

$$Recall = \frac{TN}{TN + FP} \qquad \text{Eq. (3.12)}$$

$$F1 - score = 2 \times \frac{Precision \times Recall}{Precision + Recall} \qquad \text{Eq. (3.13)}$$

The performance measures (accuracy, precision, recall, and f1-score) were evaluated to the representative ML method, including KNN, Naïve Bayes, SVM, decision tree, and the ensemble method RF algorithm. The performance result for all algorithms is shown in Table 3.2.

Furthermore, the computational time for constructing the classifier model of the representative ML algorithms is shown in Figure 3.7.

**Table 3.2**  Result Performance of Classifier Models

| MODEL | ACCURACY | RECALL | PRECISION | F1-SCORE |
|---|---|---|---|---|
| DecisionTreeClassifier | 0.92 | 0.91 | 0.89 | 0.90 |
| KNeighborsClassifier | 0.93 | 0.95 | 0.89 | 0.92 |
| GaussianNB | 0.90 | 0.87 | 0.92 | 0.89 |
| SVC | 0.95 | 0.98 | 0.91 | 0.94 |
| RandomForestClassifier | 0.97 | 0.96 | 0.94 | 0.95 |

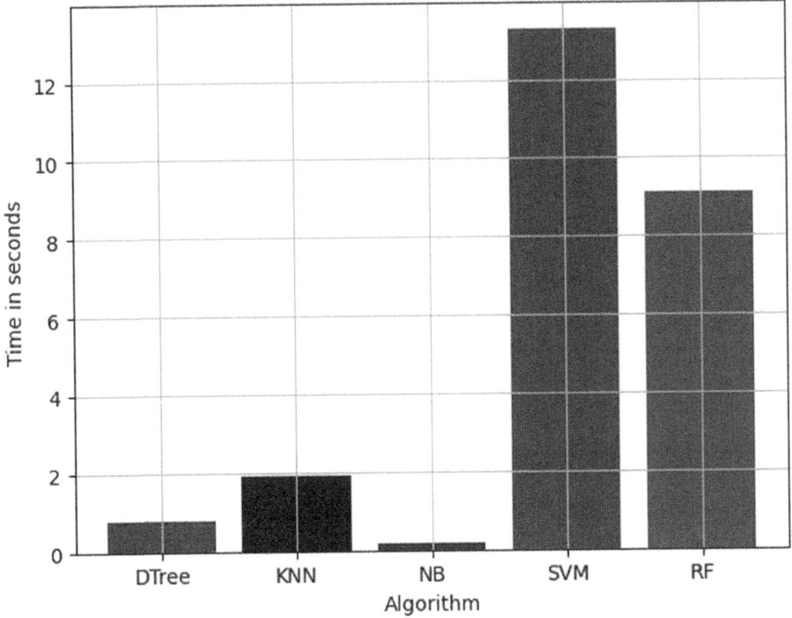


**Figure 3.7**  Comparison of computational time for the representative machine learning algorithms.

The Naïve Bayes method required the shortest time. In contrast, the longest time was required for SVM with the RBF algorithm.

## 3.7 Conclusion

The research pertaining to the identification of artemisinin drug resistance successfully implemented several ML algorithms, namely KNN, Naïve Bayes, decision tree C4.5, SVM, and RF. DNA barcode sequences comprised the dataset, which was encoded prior to its application to the classifier model for detection purposes. In general, the algorithms demonstrated exceptional f1-score performance.

The RF algorithm demonstrated the most optimal performance in terms of f1-score, recall, and accuracy. The computational time required by RF is considerable.

## 3.8 Future Work

Research related to the prediction of artemisinin drug resistance has been implemented using ML. Therefore, it can be further developed for other anti-malarial drugs. Modelling with RF has achieved a high level of performance, but it also requires significant computational time. This is due to the precise combination of parameters for that method. Hence, development related to hyperparameter optimization is needed.

### Acknowledgement

This research was financially supported by Faculty of Computer Science, Brawijaya University on a program of Doctoral Associate Professor Grant in 2022 under contract number: DIPA- FILKOM-3511-1/2022-1 dated on January 4, 2022.

# Reference


1. S. J. Patgiri *et al.*, "Characterization of Drug Resistance and Genetic Diversity of Plasmodium Falciparum Parasites from Tripura, Northeast India," *Sci Rep, Vol.* 9, no. 1, p. 13704, Dec. 2019, doi: 10.1038/s41598-019-50152-w.
2. L. Cui, S. Mharakurwa, D. Ndiaye, P. K. Rathod and P. J. Rosenthal, "Antimalarial Drug Resistance: Literature Review and Activities and Findings of the ICEMR Network," *Am J Trop Med Hyg*, vol. 93, no. 3 Suppl, pp. 57–68, 2015, doi: 10.4269/ajtmh.15-0007.
3. J.-J. Wilson, K.-W. Sing, and N. Jaturas, "DNA Barcoding: Bioinformatics Workflows for Beginners," in *Encyclopedia of Bioinformatics and Computational Biology*, S. Ranganathan, M. Gribskov, K. Nakai, and C. Schönbach, Eds., Oxford: Academic Press, 2019, pp. 985–995. doi: 10.1016/B978-0-12-809633-8.20468-8.
4. L. Adlung, Y. Cohen, U. Mor and E. Elinav, "Machine Learning in Clinical Decision Making," *Med*, vol. 2, no. 6, pp. 642–665, 2021, doi: 10.1016/j.medj.2021.04.006.
5. N. Ali, D. Neagu and P. Trundle, "Evaluation of k-Nearest Neighbour Classifier Performance for Heterogeneous Data Sets," *SN Appl Sci*, vol. 1, no. 12, p. 1559, 2019, doi: 10.1007/s42452-019-1356-9.

6. N. P. Aprilia, D. Pratiwi and A. B. Ariwibowo, "Sentiment Visualization of Covid-19 Vaccine Based on Naive Bayes Analysis," *J Inf Technol Comput Sci*, vol. 6, no. 2, Art. no. 2, Oct. 2021, https://jitecs.ub.ac.id/index.php/jitecs/article/view/353

7. A. R. Isnain, J. Supriyanto and M. P. Kharisma, "Implementation of K-Nearest Neighbor (K-NN) Algorithm for Public Sentiment Analysis of Online Learning," *Indonesian J Comput Cybern Sys*, vol. 15, no. 2, Art. no. 2, Apr. 2021, doi: 10.22146/ijccs.65176.

8. A. V. Ullal and R. Weissleder, "Photocleavable DNA Barcoding Antibodies for Multiplexed Protein Analysis in Single Cells," *Methods Mol Biol*, vol. 1346, pp. 47–54, 2015, doi: 10.1007/978-1-4939-2987-0_4.

9. T. M. Mitchell, *Machine Learning*. in McGraw-Hill series in computer science. New York: McGraw-Hill, 1997.

10. O. Sutton, "Introduction to k nearest neighbour classification and condensed nearest neighbour data reduction," *University lectures, University of Leicester*, vol. 1, 2012.

11. A. W. S. B. Johan, F. Utaminingrum and A. S. Budi, "K-Value Effect for Detecting Stairs Descent Using Combination GLCM and KNN," *J Inf Technol Comput Sci*, vol. 5, no. 1, pp. 23–31, 2020.

12. "Naive Bayes Classifier - an overview | ScienceDirect Topics." Accessed: Nov. 26, 2020. [Online]. Available: https://www.sciencedirect.com/topics/engineering/naive-bayes-classifier

13. L. Zhang, L. Luo, L. Hu and M. Sun, "An SVM-Based Classification Model for Migration Prediction of Beijing.," *Eng Lett*, vol. 28, no. 4, 2020.

14. W. F. S. Auliya, Y. A. Mahmudy, "Land Clustering for Potato Plants Using Hybrid Particle Swarm Optimization and K-Means Improved by Random Injection," *J Inf Technol Comput Sci*, vol. 4, no. 1, pp. 42–56, 2019.

15. A. H. Khaleel and I. Q. Abduljaleel, "A Novel Technique for Speech Encryption Based on k-Means Clustering and Quantum Chaotic Map," *Bull Electr Eng Inform*, vol. 10, no. 1, pp. 160–170, 2021.

16. M. D. R. Wahyudi, "Evaluation of TF-IDF Algorithm Weighting Scheme in The Qur'an Translation Clustering with K-Means Algorithm," *J Inf Technol Comput Sci*, vol. 6, no. 2, pp. 117–129, 2021.

17. S. Vijayakumar and S. Wu, "Sequential Support Vector Classifiers and Regression.," in *IIA/SOCO*, 1999.

18. R. Pandya and J. Pandya, "C5. 0 Algorithm to Improved Decision Tree with Feature Selection and Reduced Error Pruning," *Int J Comput Appl*, vol. 117, no. 16, pp. 18–21, 2015.

19. U. Ojha, M. Jain, G. Jain and R. K. Tiwari, "Significance of important attributes for decision making using C5. 0," in *2017 8th International Conference on Computing, Communication and Networking Technologies (ICCCNT)*, 2017, pp. 1–4.

20. Y. Wang, Q. Han, Y. Li and Y. Li, "Video Smoke Detection Based on Multi-Feature Fusion and Modified Random Forest.," *Eng Lett*, vol. 29, no. 3, 2021.

21. N. Jiang, F. Fu, H. Zuo, X. Zheng and Q. Zheng, "A Municipal PM2. 5 Forecasting Method Based on Random Forest and WRF Model.," *Eng Lett*, vol. 28, no. 2, 2020.

22. L. Breiman, "Random Forests," *Machine Learning*, vol. 45, no. 1, pp. 5–32, 2001.

23. H. He and Y. Ma, Eds., *Imbalanced Learning: Foundations, Algorithms, and Applications*, 1st edition. Hoboken, New Jersey: Wiley-IEEE Press, 2013.

24. S. Loukas, "Multi-class Classification: Extracting Performance Metrics from the Confusion Matrix," Medium. Accessed: Mar. 06, 2022. [Online]. Available: https://towardsdatascience.com/multi-class-classification-extracting-performance-metrics-from-the-confusion-matrix-b379b427a872

4

# Cutting Edge AI

## To Build an Affordable Healthcare System

P DIVYASHREE, PRIYANKA DWIVEDI,
AND ACHINTYA KR. SARKAR

### 4.1 Introduction

Affordable healthcare for everyone is a global concern. According to the World Health Organization (WHO), about half of the world's population does not have access to healthcare services. Moreover, the healthcare expenses are too high, which leads nearly 100 million people into the economic status of poverty [1]. In most developing countries, about 75% of people live in remote villages and suffer from acute levels of poverty, unable to access the proper medical facilities for quality treatments [2]. The traditional medical sector faces many challenges such as the unavailability of infrastructure to diagnose and treat large numbers of people. The lower doctor-to-patient ratio limits access to high-quality healthcare. Transportation to reach healthcare providers from distant locations further increases the expense for patients.

The low cost and reachability of healthcare services are of major concern today. Therefore, an affordable, reliable, and uninterrupted healthcare solution for society is the pressing demand of the present day. This problem can be solved with the fusion of advanced technologies (low-cost sensors, Internet of Things [IoT] protocols, low-power computation) with artificial intelligence (AI) [3]. Cutting-edge AI algorithms have the potential to provide smart healthcare solutions with low cost and high reliability. In addition, the sensor network embedded with intelligent analysis connected with various platforms of hardware, software, smartphone apps etc., can develop and disseminate a complete end-to-end healthcare solution. Some of the advantages of an AI-based healthcare system include being operational 24/7 and not experiencing human fatigue. This system can generate an alarm in a critical observation that can be further examined by the healthcare expert (even from a remote location in real-time)

DOI: 10.1201/9781032667508-4

**49**

for correct decision-making. In this way, AI-based healthcare systems can provide quality health services to a large population from a remote location at an affordable cost.

Many efforts have been made in the literature to develop an affordable healthcare system by developing low-cost sensors, better Machine Learning (ML) algorithms, and protocols for data privacy and transmission. Garbhapu et al. [4] developed a low-cost wristband-based biomedical wearable healthcare system. The wristbands were incorporated with a pulse oximeter and temperature sensors to collect the vital signs of many people at the same time and communicate the information to the remote doctor or healthcare facility. The entire prototype consisted of low-cost system components such as the sensor hub, microcontroller MSP430G2553, wireless transmitter nRF24L01, IEEE 802.14.4, and a Raspberry Pi 3. Therefore, the proposed system provides an economic healthcare solution to a large-scale population. A smart healthcare system comprises several components such as sensors, IoT, AI, communication protocol, computational resources, and smart apps. Cost-effectiveness can be achieved with the development of low-cost system components. Sensors are one of the major components of a healthcare system, and the development of low-cost and precision sensors can significantly reduce its cost. The reduction in cost makes it economically feasible for real-life implementation. Recently, technological innovations in low-cost sensing devices such as paper-based flexible sensors and wearable healthcare devices [5–8] created the primary path toward the reduction of sensor cost. The availability of popular open-source toolkits for building AI algorithms such as Scikit[1], TensorFlow[2], and PyTorch[3] and advanced communication protocols such as 5G and 6G will help in the transmission of healthcare information at a faster pace. In addition, sensing, actuation, and medical data interpretation in the interconnected system is important for providing real-time smart solutions in the healthcare industry. These have become feasible with the advancement of integrated circuit (IC) technology i.e., sensor design. The technology of fog computing has a major role in smart healthcare that reduces the computation burden of cloud servers. Thus, cost-effective real-time healthcare data analysis is possible [9]. Smart apps with data encryption technology will communicate healthcare data to concerned persons not only at a faster speed using high-tech communication protocols but also in

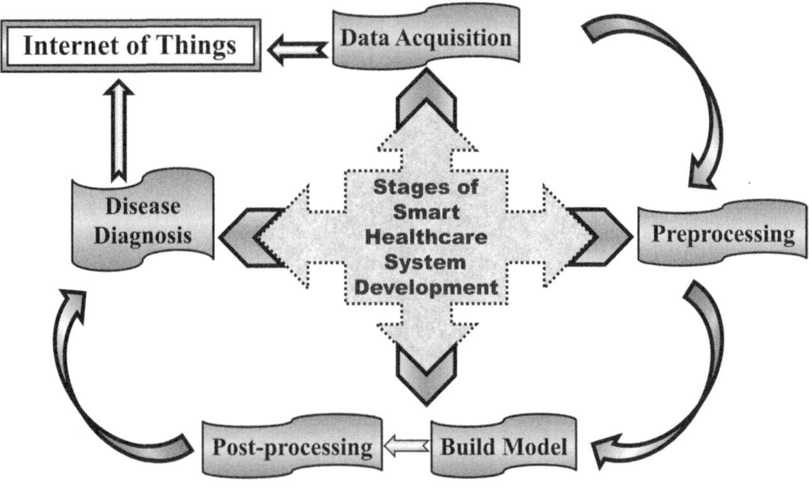



**Figure 4.1**   Stages of developing a smart healthcare system.

a reliable and trustworthy way. Ambient assisted living is one of the revolutions in healthcare wherein robots assist patients in their daily activities and act as companions for the elderly to help overcome their loneliness.

Overall, the integration of technologies like miniaturized sensors, IoT, wireless communication, and AI can provide continuous and reliable services at an affordable cost [10]. Typically, there are various stages in the realization of a smart healthcare system as shown in Figure 4.1.

In Figure 4.1, the sensor network continuously collects biosignal data from humans. This data is preprocessed (e.g. artifact removal, feature extraction for useful representation) and then fed to the AI algorithms to learn the attributes related to the application (called the model) in the training phase. The model obtained during training is used for diagnosing the specific disease for a given biosignal at the test phase. All these components are integrated and communicated using an IoT interface.

## 4.2 The Path toward Achieving Affordable Healthcare

This section briefly presents the various advancements in technologies for the development of affordable smart healthcare systems, a few case studies on breast cancer classification using chest mammography, renal tumor detection using multiphase computed tomography (CT) scans, and smart healthcare systems using smart-watches. Further, the advancement in sensor technology for low-cost healthcare sensors will be discussed comprehensively. For the development of a low-cost smart healthcare system with AI, the medical database is a key factor in learning the AI algorithm. Table 4.1 shows different databases available freely to the research community to develop an AI-based disease-diagnostic healthcare system.

To understand the role of AI in the healthcare sector and have insight into the AI-based healthcare system, a few case studies are described below.

### 4.2.1  *Case Study 1: Breast Cancer Detection Using the Mammogram Image*

Figure 4.2 illustrates the entire flow of classifying the normal and breast cancer types of malignant and benign conditions using mammograms of the chest [31]. The database comprises 95 mammogram images (including malignant, benign, and normal patients) of the chest.

The mammogram images were first preprocessed to remove the muscle images, which are not very close in intensity to a tumor image, with a segmentation technique based on maximum likelihood condition. Next, the two-dimensional Hough transform is applied to find arbitrary shapes in the image to detect the abnormality.

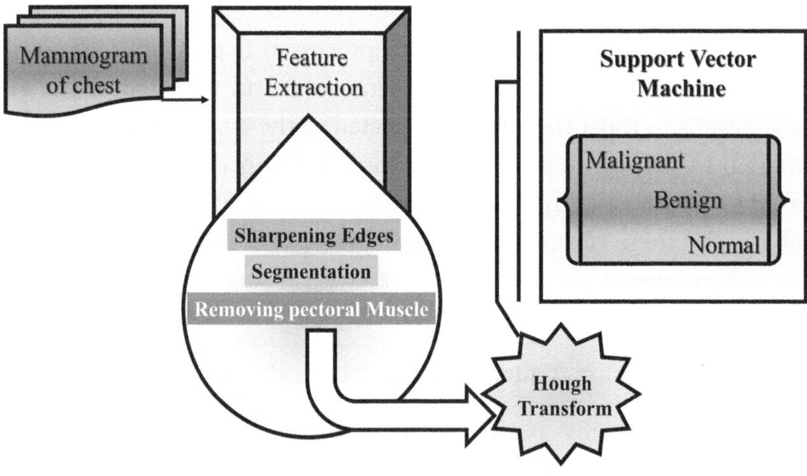


**Figure 4.2**   Breast cancer classification using support vector machine.

**Table 4.1** Medical Database Available Free of Cost

| S/ NO. | DATABASE | INFORMATION ABOUT DATA | META DATA |
|---|---|---|---|
| 1 | Breast cancer Database [11] | Gene, protein, and drug | 1. Gene ID, gene name, gene type, gene symbol, organism, taxonomic lineage, gene function, proteins coded by the gene, and gene description.<br>2. Protein information in FASTA format.<br>3. Drug ID, drug bank ID, drug name, drug category, IUPAC name, molecular weight, action, description, logP value, indication, pharmacology, toxicity, protein binding, and biotransformation. |
| 2 | PLCO database [12] | Prostate, lung, colorectal, and ovarian | 155,000 participants' cancer data |
| 3 | Adult Cardiac Surgery Database [13] | Cardiac surgery procedure record | 7.5 million cardiac surgery process, consists of 3800 participating physicians, anesthesiologists, and surgeons |
| 4 | Abdominal and Direct Fetal Electrocardiogram (ECG) database [14] | Multichannel fetal ECG | 5 women in labor that are in the gestation period of 38 to 41 weeks |
| 5 | Arterial Fibrillation (AF) Termination Challenge Database [15] | 2 Channel ECG recordings | 20–24 hours long recording of ECG with 128 Hz frequency. Each record consists of one-minute segmentation of AF. |
| 6 | AHA Database sample excluded record [16] | 3 hours of recording of the ECG signals | 80 recordings of 2-channel analog ambulatory ECG. Sampled at 125 Hz with a resolution of 12 bits for a range of 10 mV. |
| 7 | A Large scale 12 –lead ECG database for arrhythmia study [17] | 12-lead ECG signals | 45,152 patients' ECG data. Analog/Digital (A/D) is a 4.88 V bit resolution of 32 bits. |
| 8 | A multicamera and multimodal dataset for posture and gait analysis [18] | Gait and posture | 14 healthy persons, 10 are male and 4 are female. Their weight is $69.7 \pm 11.4$ kg and height is $172 \pm 10.2$ cm with the age of $25.4 \pm 2.31$ |
| 9 | Apnea ECG Database [19] | Digital ECG | 70 records of ECG each for 10 hours duration. Set of apnea annotations derived by experts, QRS annotations, $SpO_2$, oxygen saturation respiration from the chest, abdominal, oronasal |

(Continued)

**Table 4.1**    Medical Database Available Free of Cost *(Continued)*

| S/ NO. | DATABASE | INFORMATION ABOUT DATA | META DATA |
| --- | --- | --- | --- |
| 10 | Pressure map dataset for in-bed posture classification [20] | Posture pressure data | 13 participants' pressure data in 8 standard postures and 9 additional states. 8 participants in 29 different states and 3 standard postures. The sampling rate of 1 Hz. Each file consists of about 2 minutes with 120 frames. |
| 11 | Wearable exam stress dataset for predicting cognitive performances in real-world settings [21] | Electrodermal Activity (EDA), heart rate, blood volume pulse, skin surface temperature, interbeat interval, and accelerometer data. | Subject wears an FDA-approved Empatica E4 wristband during 2 midterm and final exams. Each exam lasts 1.5 hours. Dataset includes 2 female and 8 male participants. E4 captures heart rate, body temperature, accelerometer, and skin conductance. |
| 12 | BIDMC Photoplethysmogra-phy (PPG) and respiration dataset [22] | PPG, impedance respiratory signal, ECG | 53 recordings, each of 8 minutes duration. PPG was sampled at 125 Hz. Heart rate, $SpO_2$, and respiratory rate were sampled at 1 Hz. Manual annotations of breath were included along with age and gender. |
| 13 | Big IDEAs Lab glycemic variability and wearable sensor data [23] | Interstitial glucose concentration, blood volume pulse, heart rate, interbeat interval, EDA, skin temperature, and tri-axial accelerometry | 16 patients wear emphatic E4 and Dexcom G6 wrist-worn devices for 8–10 days. The sampling rate of PPG was 64 Hz, accelerometry was 32 Hz, EDA and skin temperature were 4 Hz. |
| 14 | Electroencephalogram (EEG) motor movement/ Imagery dataset [24] | 64-channel EEG recording | 1500 records of 1–2-minute EEG recordings from 109 volunteers. EEG signals were captured for eyes being open, closed, open and close or right fist, imagining opening and closing left or right fist, opening and closing fists or both feet, imagine opening and closing both fists or feet. |

*(Continued)*

**Table 4.1**  Medical Database Available Free of Cost *(Continued)*

| S/ NO. | DATABASE | INFORMATION ABOUT DATA | META DATA |
|---|---|---|---|
| 15 | EEG during mental arithmetic tasks [25] | 23-channel EEG recorded during mental arithmetic tasks | Used XAI-MEDICA EEG sensor to collect signals while performing mental arithmetic operations. |
| 16 | EEG signals from Rapid Serial Visualization Presentation (RSVP) [26] | 8-channel EEG | EEG data from 11 patients collected from scalp channel locations of PO8, PO7, PO3, PO4, P7, P8, O1, and O2 was collected during RSVP. |
| 17 | Effect of deep brain stimulation on Parkinsonian Tremor [27] | Rest tremor velocity of Parkinson disease affected people | 16 subjects' data was collected, 11 are male and 5 are female. |
| 18 | MIMIC database [28] | Bedside data of ECG and clinical data from medical records | 90 Intensive Care Unit (ICU) patients' data for 20–40 hours or more. Annotation labels are given to ECG beats. |
| 19 | EDA of healthy volunteers [29] | EDA | EDA at rest and awake conditions were collected from 11 healthy persons. |
| 20 | HiRID, a high time-resolution ICU dataset [30] | Monitoring of ICU patients | 34,000 patients' data of demography, bedside monitoring data, measurements and settings of mechanical ventilation, observation of healthcare providers, lab values and suggested drugs, and fluid and nutrition data. |

The Hough-transformed images are then used to extract intensity features, including mean, variance, entropy, and standard deviation. The extracted features are used to classify normal and abnormal (breast cancer types—benign and malignant) using SVM. This SVM-based system yields an accuracy of 94% in breast cancer classification [31].

### 4.2.2 Case Study 2: End-to-End Deep Learning Techniques for Kidney Cancer Diagnosis

Recently, bioinspired deep neural network (DNN)-based ML has emerged as a reliable modeling technique in various domains including healthcare services. Figure 4.3 illustrates a kidney cancer diagnosis system using convolutional neural networks (CNN). In this system, 1035 multiphase CT images from 308 patients who underwent renal tumor surgery from 2003 to 2020 were considered. The dataset consists of images from five major renal tumors: oncocytoma, acute myeloid leukemia (AML), chromophobe renal cell carcinoma (chRCC), papillary renal cell carcinoma (pRCC), and clear cell renal cell carcinoma (ccRCC).

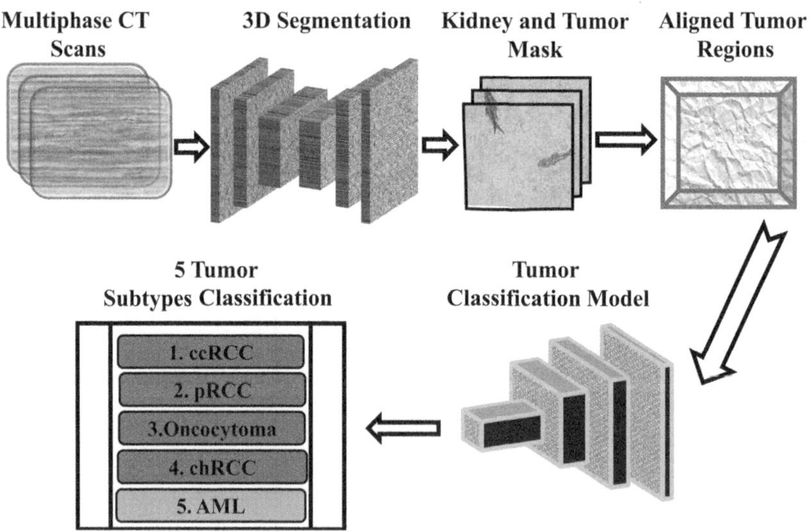


**Figure 4.3**   Automated diagnosis of subtypes in renal tumors using deep neural network techniques.

For system evaluation, 50 images are randomly selected and the rest are considered for training. The multiphase CT scan images are then input into the system and a three-dimensional (3D) CNN U-Net model is applied at the segmentation step for extracting the kidney and tumor masks. Subsequently, the alignment of the tumor regions across the different phases is detected. Further, the aligned tumor region is fed into a CNN to classify the five tumor types at the output layers using the cross-entropy-based objective function [32]. The choice of 3D U-Net for segmentation was made in the system because it outperformed compared to the baseline models for kidney tumor segmentation as per the KiTS19 challenge [33]. The system was developed using the PyTorch framework and executed in an Nvidia Titan Xp Graphics Processing Unit (GPU). This system was able to predict/diagnose the correct subtype of the renal tumor with 75% accuracy [32].

### 4.2.3 Case Study 3: A Smart Wearable Healthcare System for Monitoring Health Issues

A smart wearable healthcare system involves the integration of wearable sensors, smartphones, communication interfaces, and storage. Technology is a boon but also has its challenges for real-world implementation. For instance, if there is a network problem, data cannot be transmitted to the cloud, which may become an emergency since the acquisition of data at the right time is critical in making decisions on treatment. To address this issue, Kartikasari et al. [34] proposed a store-forward method with a buffer unit for uninterrupted data transfer in smart healthcare. Figure 4.4 shows a smart wearable healthcare system architecture with reliable data transmission. The system comprises a smart watch embedded with sensors (gyroscope, heart rate, and accelerometer) to monitor health. The smartwatch includes a smartOS protocol for the collection and transmission of vital signals. The Bluetooth and Wi-Fi connection communicate the information between a smartwatch, smartphone, and cloud storage. The smartphone is equipped with a buffer that provides delay tolerance in case data acquisition is stopped because of network failure. The major objective of this work was to have temporary storage that has the capability to handle 30 minutes of network discontinuity. All these

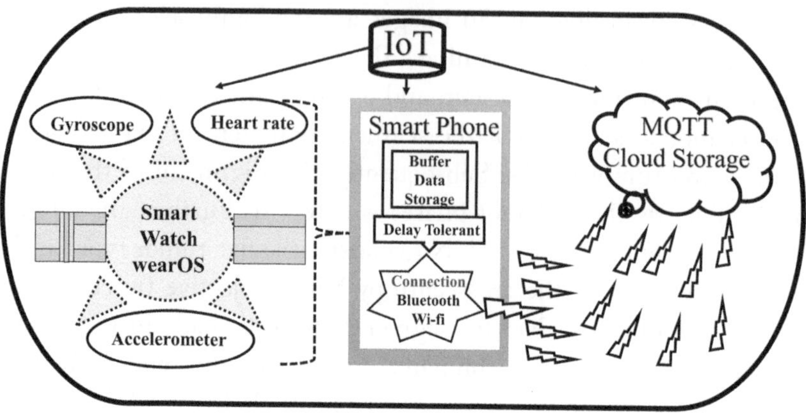


**Figure 4.4** Architecture of store-forward smart healthcare system for reliable healthcare services.

system components are connected through a lightweight MQTT IoT-based framework.

With the incorporation of AI, cost minimization in healthcare services can be achieved. Therefore, knowledge of AI and its model architecture is essential in building a cost-effective healthcare system. For healthcare prediction purposes, these algorithms can be employed based on their relevance to the application. The early diagnosis of the disease is possible with the computational analysis of medical data. This early prediction helps in the minimization of the diagnosis and treatment cost at the later stages. The danger of the disease progressing to extreme stages can be reduced by taking precautionary measures to avoid late disease diagnosis and high treatment costs. Disease progression can be monitored and relevant measures can be taken. All these healthcare solutions are achievable through AI advancements. There are many algorithms in the realm of AI. AI can be broadly categorized into ML-based algorithms and Deep Learning (DL)-based algorithms. Some of the current supervised ML algorithms are K-Nearest Neighbor, support vector machines, decision trees, classification and regression trees, logistic regression, Random Forest, Naive Bayes, and artificial neural networks. The unsupervised ML algorithms include partition clustering, graph-based clustering, hierarchical clustering, density-based clustering, model-based clustering, semi-supervised learning, evolutionary learning, and active learning [35]. A few of the DL models include CNNs, recurrent neural networks, deep belief networks, and stacked encoders. The hybrid model is a combination of different algorithms that can improve the performance of disease diagnosis. The AI models assist in making healthcare decisions such as disease identification or classification, drug delivery, treatment planning etc. Therefore, robust healthcare solutions can be provided to large-scale sectors at a reliable cost [36].

### 4.2.4 Sensor Technology Advancement for Low-Cost Healthcare

This subsection describes the role of wearable sensor technology and digital diagnosis in building cost-effective smart healthcare systems. As the main objective is to build an affordable healthcare system/solution and the sensor is one of the key components for sensing the signals in the healthcare system. It demands a low cost (design and fabrication), reliability, and precision of the sensor. In this direction, Han et al. [37] developed a low-cost plastic optical fiber sensor that was placed inside a mattresses for the continuous monitoring of sleep performance. The embedded sensor monitored respiration and heart rate during sleep. The optical fiber in the mattress responds to variations in the pressure of the body while inhaling and exhaling, leading to changes in the light intensity passing through the mattress, which quantifies breath and heart rate. Data relating to the patient lying, moving, leaving the bed, or if the person was present or not present on the bed, were captured. This data of breath and heart rate patterns analyzed the behavior and posture while sleeping. This developed a low-cost remote healthcare system that was an easily accessible and affordable solution. Also, there are significant advancements in sensor design to meet the demand of medical applications. Recently, a flexible paper-based sensor that is of low cost has been developed [8]. These sensors were fabricated on a substrate (cheap and abundantly available raw materials) that was inexpensive. The sensor is also portable and easy to operate. These features make it a viable material for paper-based sensors for use in applications such as point-of-care diagnostics under resource-poor conditions, activity monitoring etc., for large-scale utility in real-world healthcare applications [6, 7].

### 4.2.5 Digital Pathology for Affordable Remote Healthcare

The digital diagnosis, receiving expert suggestions in the diagnosis of disease, has revolutionized traditional healthcare. Through this, traveling time and expense to reach a medical specialist can be significantly reduced. This technology enables sharing of high-quality images of pathology samples across the expert group through a computer network for the diagnosis of disease. However, there are a number of challenges in digital pathology such as the data being centralized, storage crises of high-fidelity images, and network limitations in the transmission of higher-resolution digital pathology samples. To mitigate some of these issues, Subramanian et al. [38] proposed a decentralized healthcare system for data communication and storage. The proposed method provides affordable and fast healthcare solutions through digital media.

Therefore, AI and technology-assisted healthcare play a crucial role in transforming traditional nursing practices. Digital health technologies enhance the relationship between nursing staff and the patient [39]. In this way, online diagnosis and monitoring of health conditions can be developed as an affordable healthcare solution achieved through cutting-edge AI.

## 4.3  Targets for AI-assisted Healthcare Systems

One of the essentials of affordable healthcare is that the system is reliable in decision making. Due to the nature of different physiological parameters of human beings and other health-related issues, the biosignal pattern for a particular abnormality in the heart, brain etc., varies significantly across the population. Therefore, personalized healthcare is one of the most booming areas of research in recent times. Innovations in technologies have developed person-specific healthcare solutions. The textile-based sensor, wearable and skin-like sensing devices, and smart gloves embedded with sensor structures are the paths toward achieving personalized healthcare. Thus, wearable sensor technology acquires biomedical signals that can assist in the development of smart robot prosthetics. There are numerous neuromorphic prosthetics applications for personalized healthcare assistance [40], such as electrooculogram sensors placed 1 cm from the eye that will capture its movement to control a wheelchair without external efforts based on the linear discriminant analysis classifier [41]. The magnetic tracer mounted on the tongue that controls home appliances in a smart home environment provides interactive capability to severely disabled persons [42]. Temko et al. proposed a personalized diagnostic model for neonatal seizure detection. The author used an online adaptation (i.e., on-the-fly incorporation of patient-specific EEG characteristics in the model) without clinical labels. This system reduces the false detections (FD) per hour from 0.4 to 0.2 FD/h. Thus, personalized healthcare predictions were performed [43].

Complete recovery with faster treatment protocols and cost minimization is another motive for smart healthcare solutions. Thus, to quicken the recovery of patients, precision medicine is an innovation. The field of drug discovery and selectivity has emerged. AI-based big data modeling helps in the rational development of novel drugs, which provide efficient treatment to maintain public health [44, 45]. High throughput screening techniques are one of the AI innovations for the cost-effective analysis of drug discovery [46]. The expenditure for healthcare services can be drastically reduced with at-home self-care. The AI-integrated solution with a smart home enables the management of chronic diseases in the patient's own home and connects with healthcare specialists remotely. Tools, such as software, mobile applications, and smartphones, can effectively communicate the physical dynamics of patients. Thus, the patient's health condition can be effectively monitored [47]. The smart home equipped with healthcare robotics aids in remote diagnosis and treatment decisions. The sensing network comprises bed sensors, heart rate sensors, pyroelectric sensors, motion sensors, fall detection sensors, ultrasonic receivers on the ceiling, and radio frequency transmitters. These sensors will collect various signals from humans to monitor their activity. The emergence of telemedicine through multiuser telehealth kiosks and Web-based interfaces through video conferencing provides treatment suggestions remotely. AI assists in the early identification and probability of occurrence of disease, diagnosis of disease suffering, and decision-making using its wide spectrum of architectures [48]. There are various advancements in robotic infrastructure for the smart hospital such as ambulance robots, receptionist robots, nursing robots, telemedicine radiologist robots, food serving robots, outdoor delivery robots, cleaning robots, disinfectant spraying robots, surgical robots, teleoperated robots for remote operation, and rehabilitation robots [49]. For the efficient provision of healthcare services, the estimation of triage, i.e., severity-based priority [50]. The advancement in DL algorithms was used for cardiac disease diagnosis through wearable sensor networks and ambient assisted living [51].

## 4.4 Constraints in AI for Healthcare Solutions

AI algorithms suffer from a few challenges that constrain their utility in healthcare applications. A few of these limitations are discussed in this section. AI algorithms may face overfitting and under-fitting issues due to a lack of vast amounts of medical data, which limits its deployment in the real world. The limitation of data sparsity could be reduced with the help of data augmentation techniques and hyperparameter optimization [52]. The computation and power requirements are high for the complicated models, and affordability is still a challenge for implementation in real-time scenarios. The security in healthcare needs to be preserved and AI should be upgraded to meet the high-security requirements of handling medical data.

## 4.5 Future Endeavors for AI to Provide Affordable Healthcare Application

The goal for the next generation of AI-assisted healthcare is to provide reasoning for the decision it generates. Explainable AI tries to address this and provide the justification for its decision. Through reasoning, the medical expert can consider the AI-generated decision and decide the next step of medical treatment. At present, there is human intervention required to perform diagnosis and treatment. To enhance human-computer interaction and provide accurate healthcare, explainable AI plays a crucial role [53]. Federated learning is one of the technological advancements that will address the most challenging issue of healthcare data availability, preserving the security of medical information etc., in smart healthcare solutions. This pioneering technology also addresses resource optimization and reduces the computational complexity of AI models. Training a centralized model on decentralized data provides data sharing; the training brought onto the device is combined across various devices, providing diverse data-learning capabilities. Moreover, a subset of the model is selected for the training, which reduces computation resources and time to a significant level. By sharing the results only with the server and not the entire model, this reduces the storage requirement, which implies fewer data-storage resources and lower costs. The data shared is encrypted, which enhances the security of the information. The key to the encryption is not available on the server, making hacking very difficult and, thus, tightening security aspects. Therefore, secured aggregation is achieved that enables the combining of the encrypted results and decrypting only the aggregate. The zero-sum masks scramble the training results before sending them to the secured aggregate server. This ensures that the AI model performs well on an unknown dataset without overfitting the training model. Differential privacy is established to control the model memorization capability. Thus, a secured and federated AI model is trained on-device and shared across the platforms for testing. Training directly on user data without centralization is the key feature of federated learning. Distributed computing in federated learning enables the updating of models from thousands of users in the network. Collaborative learning through federated computing helps diagnose with high security and maintains the privacy of healthcare data [54]. Medical dataset availability faces many challenges; however, the collaborative learning technique in federated AI solves this issue. The federated data-driven models in a decentralized manner can be built for healthcare predictions [55]. For real-world deployment, edge devices operating with AI algorithms are required. Special architectures such as MobileNet and SqueezeNet were designed to provide computationally efficient ML models for inference on edge devices. The cluster federated learning architecture deployed on edge diagnosed COVID-19 disease in a secure way [56].

## 4.6 Conclusion

This chapter presents a comprehensive understanding of the advancements in technology and AI as the cutting-edge solution to provide affordable healthcare services to large sections of the population. The broad perspective of various essential components and a few case studies pertaining to smart healthcare systems are provided. Present-day healthcare services suffer from various challenges to meet the present-day needs. To resolve them, building an accessible and affordable healthcare system is necessary. Cutting-edge AI and allied advanced technologies, such as low-cost sensors, digital diagnosis, and robotics, play a substantial role in the realization of large-scale healthcare services. The emergence of advanced technologies with AI creates the path for automated smart healthcare solutions at an optimized price. The AI-integrated advanced technology's achievements in healthcare include real-time monitoring, seamless data sharing to medicos remotely, early diagnosis, personalized medicine, and precision healthcare. The future endeavors of incorporating explainability into AI decisions can enhance the authentication of treatment. Advanced AI algorithms such as federated learning assist in the realization of computationally efficient and low-cost models. Therefore, the intelligent integration of AI and other assistive technologies could disrupt traditional healthcare services with smart and affordable healthcare solutions.

## Notes

1  htttps://scikit-learn.org/
2  https://www.tensorflow.org/
3  https://pytorch.org/

## References


1. WHO and World Bank. (2017). World Bank and WHO: Half the world lacks access to essential health services, 100 million still pushed into extreme poverty because of health expenses. WHO. https://www.who.int/news/item/13-12-2017-world-bank-and-who-half-the-world-lacks-access-to-essential-health-services-100-million-still-pushed-into-extreme-poverty-because-of-health-expenses.
2. India Today. 75 percent of rural India survives on Rs 33 per day. from https://www.indiatoday.in/india/story/india-rural-household-650-millions-live-on-rs-33-per-day-282195-2015-07-13 (access on date).
3. Alshamrani M. (2022). IoT and Artificial Intelligence Implementations for Remote Healthcare Monitoring Systems: A Survey. Journal of King Saud University-Computer and Information Sciences, 34(8): 4687–4701. https://doi.org/10.1016/j.jksuci.2021.06.005.
4. Garbhapu V V, Gopalan S (2017) IoT Based Low Cost Single Sensor Node Remote Health Monitoring System. Procedia Computer Science, 113: 408–415, https://doi.org/10.1016/j.procs.2017.08.357.
5. Zheng Y, Tang N, Omar R, Hu Z, Duong T, Wang J, Wu W, Haick H (2021) Smart Materials Enabled with Artificial Intelligence for Healthcare Wearables. Advanced Functional Materials, 31(51): 1–20, https://doi.org/10.1002/adfm.202105482.
6. Yao Z, Coatsworth P, Shi X, Zhi J, Hu L, Yan R, Guder F, Yu H-D (2022) Paper-Based Sensors for Diagnostics, Human Activity

Monitoring, Food Safety and Environmental Detection. Sensors & Diagnostics, 1(3): 312–342, https://doi.org/10.1039/d2sd00017b.

7. Liu H, Jiang H, Du F, Zhang D, Li Z, Zhou H (2017) Flexible and Degradable Paper-Based Strain Sensor with Low Cost. ACS Sustainable Chemistry and Engineering, 5(11): 10538–10543, https://doi.org/10.1021/acssuschemeng.7b02540.

8. Jiang N, Tansukawat N D, Gonzalez-Macia L, Ates H C, Dincer C, Guder F, Tasoglu S, Yetisen A K (2021) Low-Cost Optical Assays for Point-of-Care Diagnosis in Resource-Limited Settings. ACS Sensors, 6(6): 2108–2124, https://doi.org/10.1021/acssensors.1c00669.

9. Nasr M, Islam Md M, Shehata S, Karray F, Quintana Y (2021) Smart Healthcare in the Age of AI: Recent Advances, Challenges, and Future Prospects. IEEE Access, 9: 145248–145270, https://doi.org/10.1109/ACCESS.2021.3118960.

10. Mansour R F, Amraoui A, El Nouaouri I, Diaz V G, Gupta D, Kumar S (2021) Artificial Intelligence and Internet of Things Enabled Disease Diagnosis Model for Smart Healthcare Systems. IEEE Access, 9: 45137–45146, https://doi.org/10.1109/ACCESS.2021.3066365.

11. Mohandass J, Ravichandran S, Srilakshmi K, Perumal Rajadurai C, Sanmugasamy S, Ramesh Kumar G (2010) Bioinformation BCDB-A Database for Breast Cancer Research and Information. In Bioinformation 5(1), http://www.cancer.gov/cancertopics/types/breast.

12. PLCO - The Cancer Data Access System. Retrieved October 27, 2022, from https://cdas.cancer.gov/plco/.

13. Adult Cardiac Surgery Database | STS. Retrieved October 27, 2022, from https://www.sts.org/registries/sts-national-database/adult-cardiac-surgery-database.

14. Jezewski J, Matonia A, Kupka T, Roj D, Czabanski R (2012) Abdominal and Direct Fetal ECG Database v1.0.0. Determination of the Fetal Heart Rate from Abdominal Signals: Evaluation of Beat-to-Beat Accuracy in Relation to the Direct Fetal Electrocardiogram. Biomedical Engineering/Biomedizinische Technik. https://physionet.org/content/adfecgdb/1.0.0/.

15. AF Termination Challenge Database v1.0.0. Retrieved October 27, 2022, from https://physionet.org/content/aftdb/1.0.0/.

16. AHA Database Sample Excluded Record v1.0.0. Retrieved October 27, 2022, from https://physionet.org/content/ahadb/1.0.0/.

17. Zheng J, Zhang J, Danioko S, Yao H, Guo H, Rakovski C (2020) A 12-Lead Electrocardiogram Database for Arrhythmia Research Covering More than 10,000 Patients. Scientific Data, 7(1): 48. https://doi.org/10.1038/S41597-020-0386-X.

18. A multi-camera and multimodal dataset for posture and gait analysis v1.0.0. Retrieved October 27, 2022, from https://physionet.org/content/multi-gait-posture/1.0.0/.

19. Apnea-ECG Database v1.0.0. Retrieved October 27, 2022, from https://physionet.org/content/apnea-ecg/1.0.0/.

20. A Pressure Map Dataset for In-bed Posture Classification v1.0.0. Retrieved October 28, 2022, from https://physionet.org/content/pmd/1.0.0/.

21. Rafiul Amin Md, Wickramasuriya D S, Faghih R T (2022) A Wearable Exam Stress Dataset for Predicting Grades using Physiological Signals. 2022 IEEE Healthcare Innovations and Point of Care Technologies (HI-POCT), pp 30–36, https://doi.org/10.1109/HI-POCT54491.2022.9744065.

22. BIDMC PPG and Respiration Dataset v1.0.0. Retrieved October 28, 2022, from https://physionet.org/content/bidmc/1.0.0/.

23. BIG IDEAs Lab Glycemic Variability and Wearable Device Data v1.0.0. Retrieved October 28, 2022, from https://physionet.org/content/big-ideas-glycemic-wearable/1.0.0/.

24. EEG Motor Movement/Imagery Dataset v1.0.0. Retrieved October 28, 2022, from https://physionet.org/content/eegmmidb/1.0.0/.

25. EEG During Mental Arithmetic Tasks v1.0.0. Retrieved October 28, 2022, from https://physionet.org/content/eegmat/1.0.0/.

26. EEG Signals from an RSVP Task v1.0.0. Retrieved October 28, 2022, from https://physionet.org/content/ltrsvp/1.0.0/.

27. Effect of Deep Brain Stimulation on Parkinsonian Tremor v1.0.0. Retrieved October 28, 2022, from https://physionet.org/content/tremordb/1.0.0/.

28. The MIMIC Database. Retrieved October 28, 2022, from https://archive.physionet.org/physiobank/database/mimicdb/.

29. Electrodermal Activity of Healthy Volunteers while Awake and at Rest v2.0. Retrieved October 28, 2022, from https://physionet.org/content/electrodermal-activity/2.0/.

30. HiRID, a high time-resolution ICU dataset v1.1.1. Retrieved October 28, 2022, from https://physionet.org/content/hirid/1.1.1/.

31. Vijayarajeswari R, Parthasarathy P, Vivekanandan S, Basha A A (2019) Classification of Mammogram for Early Detection of Breast Cancer Using SVM Classifier and Hough Transform. Measurement: Journal of the International Measurement Confederation, 146: 800–805, https://doi.org/10.1016/j.measurement.2019.05.083.

32. Uhm K-H, Jung S-W, Choi M H, Shin H-K, Yoo J-I, Oh S W, Kim J Y, Kim H G, Lee Y J, Youn S Y, Hong S-H, Ko S-J (2021) Deep Learning for End-to-End Kidney Cancer Diagnosis on Multi-Phase Abdominal Computed Tomography. Npj Precision Oncology, 5(1): 54, https://doi.org/10.1038/s41698-021-00195-y.

33. Heller N, Isensee F, Maier-Hein K H, Hou X, Xie C, Li F, Nan Y, Mu G, Lin Z, Han M, Yao G, Gao Y, Zhang Y, Wang Y, Hou F, Yang J, Xiong G, Tian J, Zhong C, Weight C (2021) The State of the Art in Kidney and Kidney Tumor Segmentation in Contrast-Enhanced CT Imaging: Results of the KiTS19 Challenge. Medical Image Analysis, 67: 101821, https://doi.org/10.1016/j.media.2020.101821.

34. Kartikasari D P, Tobing A, Bhawiyuga A, Kusyanti A, Purwaningtyas N H (2021) A Store-Forward Method for Biosignal Acquisition in Smart Health Care System Using Wearable IoT Device. Kinetik: Game Technology, Information System, Computer Network, Computing, Electronics, and Control, 4: 51–58, https://doi.org/10.22219/kinetik.v6i1.1154.

35. Jayatilake S M D A C, Ganegoda G U (2021) Involvement of Machine Learning Tools in Healthcare Decision Making. Journal of Healthcare Engineering, https://doi.org/10.1155/2021/6679512.

36. Shamshirband S, Fathi M, Dehzangi A, Chronopoulos A T, Alinejad-Rokny H (2021). A Review on Deep Learning Approaches in Healthcare Systems: Taxonomies, Challenges, and Open Issues. Journal of Biomedical Informatics, 113: 103627, https://doi.org/10.1016/j.jbi.2020.103627.

37. Han P, Li L, Zhang H, Guan L, Marques C, Savovic S, Ortega B, Min R, Li X (2021) Low-Cost Plastic Optical Fiber Sensor Embedded in Mattress for Sleep Performance Monitoring. Optical Fiber Technology, 64: 102541, https://doi.org/10.1016/j.yofte.2021.102541.

38. Subramanian H, Subramanian S (2022) Improving Diagnosis through Digital Pathology: Proof-of-Concept Implementation Using Smart Contracts and Decentralized File Storage. Journal of Medical Internet Research, 24(3): 1–17, https://doi.org/10.2196/34207.

39. Clancy T R (2020) Artificial Intelligence and Nursing: The Future Is Now. The Journal of Nursing Administration, 50(3): 125–127, https://doi.org/10.1097/NNA.0000000000000855.

40. Khoshmanesh F, Thurgood P, Pirogova E, Nahavandi S, Baratchi S (2021) Wearable Sensors: At the Frontier of Personalised Health Monitoring, Smart Prosthetics and Assistive Technologies. Biosensors and Bioelectronics, 176: 112946, https://doi.org/10.1016/j.bios.2020.112946.

41. Mishra S, Norton J J S, Lee Y, Lee D S, Agee N, Chen Y, Chun Y, Yeo W H (2017) Soft, Conformal Bioelectronics for a Wireless Human-Wheelchair Interface. Biosensors and Bioelectronics, 91: 796–803, https://doi.org/10.1016/j.bios.2017.01.044.

42. Krishnamurthy G, Ghovanloo M (2006) Tongue drive: a tongue operated magnetic sensor based wireless assistive technology for people with severe disabilities. IEEE International Symposium on Circuits and Systems, p 4, https://doi.org/10.1109/ISCAS.2006.1693892.

43. Temko A, Sarkar A K, Boylan G B, Mathieson S, Marnane W P, Lightbody G (2017) Toward a Personalized Real-Time Diagnosis in Neonatal Seizure Detection. IEEE Journal of Translational Engineering in Health and Medicine, 5: 1–14, https://doi.org/10.1109/JTEHM.2017.2737992.

44. Zhu H (2019) Annual Review of Pharmacology and Toxicology Big Data and Artificial Intelligence Modeling for Drug Discovery. 23(1): 1–17, https://doi.org/10.1146/annurev-pharmtox-010919.

45. Stokes J M, Yang K, Swanson K, Jin W, Cubillos-Ruiz A, Donghia N M, MacNair C R, French S, Carfrae L A, Bloom-Ackerman Z, Tran V M, Chiappino-Pepe A, Badran A H, Andrews I W, Chory E J, Church G M, Brown E D, Jaakkola T S, Barzilay R, Collins J J (2020) A Deep Learning Approach to Antibiotic Discovery. Cell, 180(4): 688–702.e13, https://doi.org/10.1016/j.cell.2020.01.021.

46. Zhang L, Tan J, Han D, Zhu H (2017) From Machine Learning to Deep Learning: Progress in Machine Intelligence for Rational Drug Discovery. Drug Discovery Today, 22(11): 1680–1685, https://doi.org/10.1016/j.drudis.2017.08.010.

47. Roy S, Singh A, Choudhary C (2021) Artificial Intelligence in Healthcare. In Lecture Notes in Networks and Systems 190, https://doi.org/10.1007/978-981-16-0882-7_24.

48. Hasan Sapci A, Aylin Sapci H (2019). Innovative Assisted Living Tools, Remote Monitoring Technologies, Artificial Intelligence-Driven Solutions, and Robotic Systems for Aging Societies: Systematic Review. JMIR Aging, 2(2): 1–16, https://doi.org/10.2196/15429.

49. Khan Z H, Siddique A, Lee C W (2020) Robotics Utilization for Healthcare Digitization in Global COVID-19 Management. International Journal of Environmental Research and Public Health, 17(11): 3819, https://doi.org/10.3390/ijerph17113819.

50. Tsumura R, Hardin J W, Bimbraw K, Grossestreuer A V, Odusanya O S, Zheng Y, Hill J C, Hoffmann B, Soboyejo W, Zhang H K (2021) Tele-Operative Low-Cost Robotic Lung Ultrasound Scanning Platform for Triage of COVID-19 Patients. IEEE Robotics and Automation Letters, 6(3): 4664–4671, https://doi.org/10.1109/LRA.2021.3068702.

51. Qureshi M A, Qureshi K N, Jeon G, Piccialli F (2022) Deep Learning-Based Ambient Assisted Living for Self-Management of Cardiovascular Conditions. Neural Computing and Applications, 34(13): 10449–10467, https://doi.org/10.1007/s00521-020-05678-w.

52. Monshi M M A, Poon J, Chung V, Monshi F M (2021) CovidXrayNet: Optimizing Data Augmentation and CNN Hyperparameters for Improved COVID-19 Detection from CXR. Computers in Biology and Medicine, 133: 104375, https://doi.org/10.1016/j.compbiomed.2021.104375.

53. Nazar M, Alam M M, Yafi E, Su'ud M M (2021) A Systematic Review of Human–Computer Interaction and Explainable Artificial Intelligence in Healthcare With Artificial Intelligence Techniques. IEEE Access, 9: 153316–153348, https://doi.org/10.1109/ACCESS.2021.3127881.

54. Yang Q, Liu Y, Cheng Y, Kang Y, Chen T, Yu H (2020) Federated Learning. In Federated Learning. Springer International Publishing, https://doi.org/10.1007/978-3-031-01585-4.

55. Rieke N, Hancox J, Li W, Milletari F, Roth H R, Albarqouni S, Bakas S, Galtier M N, Landman B A, Maier-Hein K, Ourselin S, Sheller M, Summers R M, Trask A, Xu D, Baust M, Cardoso M J (2020) The Future of Digital Health with Federated Learning. Npj Digital Medicine, 3(1): 119, https://doi.org/10.1038/s41746-020-00323-1.

56. Qayyum A, Ahmad K, Ahsan M A, Al-Fuqaha A, Qadir J (2022) Collaborative Federated Learning for Healthcare: Multi-Modal COVID-19 Diagnosis at the Edge. IEEE Open Journal of the Computer Society, 3: 172–184, https://doi.org/10.1109/ojcs.2022.3206407.

# 5

# SKIN DISEASE PREDICTION USING HYBRID CUCKOO SEARCH OPTIMIZATION WITH A SUPPORT VECTOR MACHINE ALGORITHM


SIVANANTHAM K AND
BLESSINGTON PRAVEEN P


## 5.1 Introduction

### 5.1.1 Human Skin

The skin is the largest organ in the body. It offers defence from heat, sunburn, harm, and illness. Additionally, skin regulates body temperature and stores vitamin D, water, and fat.

*5.1.1.1 Types of Skin* The two primary types of human skin are seen in Figure 5.1. One type is glabrous skin (non-hairy skin), which is constantly present on the palms and soles alternated with ridges and sulci to form grooves on its surface. These grooves have individual configurations known as dermatoglyphics. The second form is the hair-bearing skin, which lacks encapsulated sensory organs but has both hair follicles and sebaceous glands. The varieties of skin on various areas of the body also vary greatly.

*5.1.1.2 Layers of Human Skin* Figure 5.2 illustrates the three layers that make up the majority of skin, which:

- Protect against infection and serves as a waterproofing layer.
- Includes the dermis, which houses the skin's protrusions, such as the hair follicles, sweat glands, and sebaceous glands.

*5.1.1.3 Skin Cancer* The skin is made up of small building blocks called cells, much like all other human components. These cells can

DOI: 10.1201/9781032667508-5

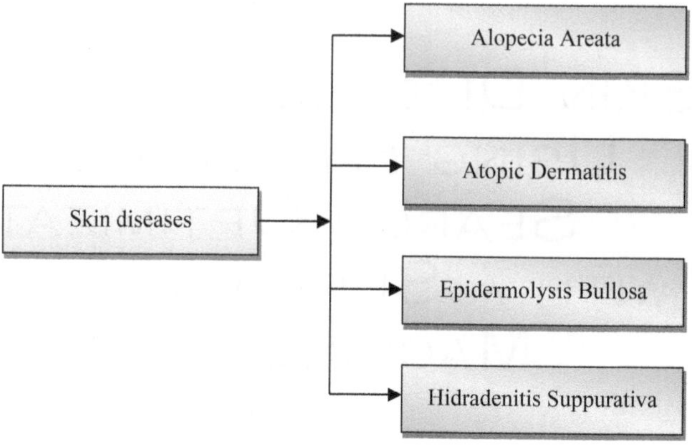



**Figure 5.1**    Four skin diseases of human skin.

occasionally develop cancer due to ultraviolet (UV) radiation exposure or other factors, such as family history. Skin growths that are abnormal might be classified as benign (not cancerous) or malignant (cancerous). Malignant growths are much more dangerous than benign growths. Moles and other benign growths are typically treatable, do not recur, and seldom pose a threat to life. Because they do not infiltrate nearby tissues, benign tumours do not disseminate to other body parts. Malignant growths, on the other hand, may be life threatening, including melanoma, basal cell cancer, and squamous cell cancer (Lu et al., 2013b). Even after being removed, they can regenerate. They may spread to other body regions because of their inclination to invade and harm organs and tissues. Basal cell cancer, squamous cell cancer, and melanocytes are three separate cell types that are present in the very top layer of the skin.

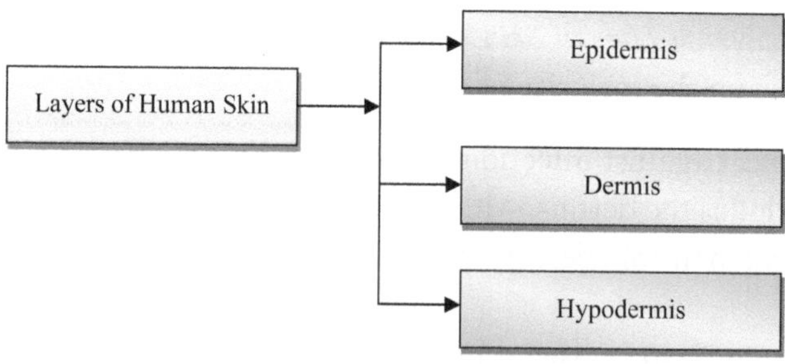



**Figure 5.2**    Layers of human skin.

*Melanoma—skin cancer:* this may not be cured if neglected; the majority of melanomas eventually spread to other regions of the body (Arivoli et al., 2015). Most cases of melanoma can be successfully treated with early discovery and surgery to remove the tumour; however, it is rarely treatable in its advanced stages. Melanoma incidence varies widely around the globe, with Australia, the United States, Norway, Switzerland, Sweden, Denmark, and Israel having the greatest incidence and Japan, the Philippines, China, and India having the lowest incidence.

Melanocytes, which make up the skin's outer layer, are where melanoma develops (Kanagaraj et al., 2014). Melanocytes generate melanin, a pigment that gives skin its tan or brown hue and aids in shielding the skin's deeper layers from the sun's harmful rays. When melanocytes undergo malignant transformation, become aberrant, proliferate out of control, and aggressively infiltrate surrounding tissues, melanoma develops (Lu et al., 2013a).

Melanoma can simply affect the skin, or it can travel through the blood or lymphatic system to other organs and bones. Any part of the skin's surface might develop melanoma. Melanoma is rare in those with dark skin. The skin on the head, neck, lower thighs, soles of the feet, palms of the hands, and under the fingernails can all exhibit it.

*Basal cell skin cancer:* The basal cell layer of the skin is where basal cell skin cancer begins. Typically, it occurs in places where repeated sun exposure has been present. For fair-skinned individuals, basal cell skin cancer is the most prevalent kind.

*Squamous cell skin cancer:* The cells that originate with squamous cell skin cancer typically occur in persons of colour, usually on bodily regions that are not exposed to sunlight, such as legs or feet. According to earlier studies, the likelihood of successfully treating cancer depends on when it is discovered. If it is not discovered early, the likelihood of success is less than 50%.

*5.1.1.4 Data Mining* Today, every person and organization, whether it be a family, business, or other organization all have access to a wealth of information about themselves and their surroundings. The potential of this data to forecast the development of intriguing factors or trends in the external environment has not yet been fully realized. Tajeripour et al. (2012) discuss two key issues. Data is inefficient since it is dispersed over numerous archive systems that are disconnected from one another. The potential for information elaboration using statistical tools is hindered because of this and obstructs the creation of effective and pertinent data synthesis. These issues might be solved by two advancements. First, as hardware and software continue to advance and become more powerful while remaining more affordable, companies can now gather and arrange data in ways that make it easier to access and share.

Second, methodological research has lately resulted in the creation of adaptable the processes can be utilized to assess enormous data stores, notably in the fields of computers and statistics (Tymińska et al., 2013). Due to these two advancements, data mining is quickly becoming a crucial intelligence tool for decision-making in many industries. Data mining aims to access massive amounts of data. This chapter discusses the stages of data up until analysis, analysis techniques, and how they are used with medical data. Data mining is covered in the first section, while medical data mining is covered in the second section.

Listed here is an illustration of the knowledge-discovery process, including the steps in an iterative sequence:

1. Cleaning of data.
2. Integration of data (where it may be integrated from several data sources).
3. Data choice (wherein the database is searched for pertinent information).
4. Data transformation (for instance, using summary or aggregate operations Figure 5.3).
5. Data mining.
6. Pattern assessment (to determine the data's most fascinating patterns using metrics).
7. Knowledge presentation, which involves using techniques for knowledge visualization and representation, are used to display mined knowledge to the user.

This chapter is arranged in five parts. Section 5.2 explains the present method and the drawback of its techniques in skin-diseases detection and segmentation. The strategies for skin-disease prediction proposed in Section 5.3 are more effective. Section 5.4 presents the

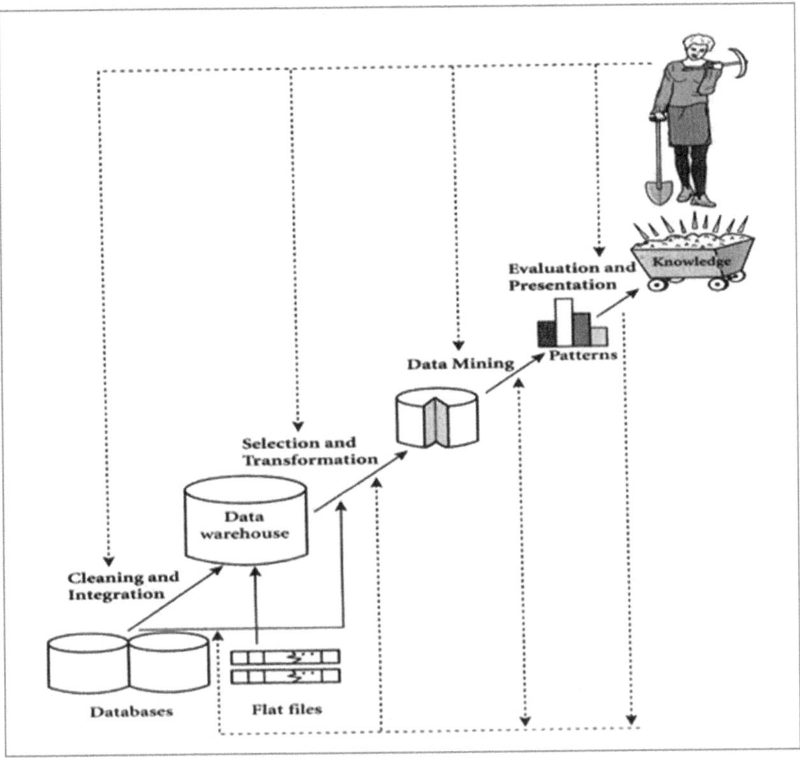


**Figure 5.3**  Data mining as a stage of the knowledge-discovery process.

experimental findings from testing on the images and their analysis, and Section 5.5 provides a conclusion.

## 5.2  Literature Review

Using the predicted depth derived from common dermoscopic pictures, a method for reconstructing a three-dimensional (3D) skin lesion is provided (Srivastava et al., 2013). The 3D reconstruction is used to extract 3D form and depth data. Regular colour, texture, and two-dimensional (2D) shape aspects are also extracted in addition to 3D data. It is essential to conduct feature extraction to get correct results. In addition to melanoma, basal cell carcinoma, blue nevus, derma-tofibroma, haemangioma, seborrhoea keratoses, and common mole lesions are among the conditions that the *in situ* melanoma system is intended to detect. Performance is assessed while taking considering various feature set combinations. Following the addition of estimated depth and 3D features, significant performance increase was noted.

Dermoscopic photographs of the cutaneous vasculature used a novel framework that has been proposed, and extracted vascular characteristics were investigated for the classification of skin cancer (Kumar et al., 2010). We divided the lesion's vascular structure into independent component analysis to break the image down into portions that represent the melanin. By doing this, the impact of pigmentation on blood vessel visibility is eliminated. Extracted vascular characteristics that divided the lesion's vascular structure were investigated for the classification of skin cancer.

Porter et al. (2011) suggested that computer-aided diagnosis (CAD) tools can be beneficial to dermatologists to facilitate the early diagnosis of malignancies because they provide a cutting-edge technique for melanoma skin-cancer detection. In the pre-processing step, images were subjected to a bank of directional filters to identify hair and other types of noise; as a consequence, an image-in-painting technique was employed to fill in the blank spaces. The lesion region border was marked on the pictures using fuzzy Markov Random Field and C-Means techniques. The technique was tested on a dataset of 200 dermoscopic images and produced superior outcomes than competing techniques.

Barati et al. (2011) suggested popular machine learning methods with accurate classification abilities include support vector machines (SVMs), which can create a real-time embedded classifier that may be applied to a low-cost portable device that is only meant for the early diagnosis of melanoma. SVM classifiers implemented in hardware for real-time applications can increase computing speed and reduce power consumption. The system technology for online melanoma classification with a field programmable gate array (FPGA)-implemented linear binary SVM classifier was displayed. The system was developed on the most recent high-level synthesis design approach and implemented on a recent hybrid platform. The system's implementation displayed great performance, sparse use of hardware resources, and minimal power consumption, all of which satisfy crucial embedded systems criteria.

Patnaik et al. (2018) suggested that it is crucial to correctly segment skin cancer photos to accurately identify the lesion region. Accurate segmentation has a significant impact on the subsequent diagnostic steps. In this paper, a technique for extracting the lesion location from digital clinical photos was suggested. It is based on deep convolutional neural networks (CNN). To reduce noise, an edge-preserving smoothing guided filter is first applied to all input images as part of the pre-processing stage. The pre-processed image is then supplied to a CNN with each pixel as the patch's centre with local and global features surrounding each pixel and are input into a CNN. The middle pixel of the patch is labelled as the CNN's output. The proposed CNN structure and pre-processing filter were ideal for this crucial segmentation operation.

A non-invasive a real-time automated system for analyzing skin lesions used to detect and prevent melanoma proposed two key elements (Chaurasia et al., 2019). First, a real-time notification alerts users before they become sunburned; this introduces a new equation for calculating when skin will burn. Second, a module was designed for automated image analysis that performs picture acquisition, hair recognition and exclusion, lesion segmentation, feature extraction, and classification. The suggested method utilizes for testing and research purposes the PH2 dermoscopy picture database from Pedro Hispano Hospital.

Verma et al. (2019) suggested that a crucial step in image analysis of pigmented skin lesions was automatic lesion segmentation. The creation of CAD systems for dermoscopic pictures is currently of great interest. One of the most crucial steps is segmentation, as the accuracy of this stage decides whether a CAD system will ultimately succeed or fail. This work presented a novel approach to segmenting dermoscopic pictures. The pre-processing step involved filtering the dermoscopy image to eliminate the majority of obstacles to accurate segmentation, such as a diversity of lesion sizes, colours, forms, and textures, as well as the presence of hairs based primarily on histogram thresholding and segmentation. Using mathematical morphology, the image was improved to provide superior segmentation with a smooth border and no noise in the lesion zone. The approach technique was assessed using the True Detection Rate (TDR) and the Hammoude Distance (HM).

Elngar et al. (2021) developed a method as computer-vision-based diagnosis tools were being employed in a number of hospitals and dermatological offices, mostly to identify malignant melanoma tumours and diagnose skin cancer early. The installation, the visual features applied to the types of skin lesions, and the methods utilized to define them were first presented in this study to assess the most recent technology for such systems. Following that, the most widely used methods for classifying skin lesions as well as employing digital image processing methods like segmentation, border detection, colour, and texture processing, how to extract these features were explained. Reporting the statistical outcomes of significant implementations that are known to exist in the literature, the paper analyses the effectiveness of many classifiers on specific skin-lesion diagnosis.

Given the high expense of treatment and mortality rate for this malignancy, early detection is promoted despite its ongoing global rise (Parikh et al., 2016). The various parts of an automated skin-cancer diagnosis include a system for automatically classifying skin cancer, as well as research into the interaction between skin-cancer images and various types of neural networks and pre-processing. The system receives the collected images and uses various image processing techniques to improve the image attributes. Region growth and merging is the foundation of the statistical region merging (SRM) algorithm. After the healthy skin has been recognized, the cancer cell is excised from the skin's afflicted area but is still visible in the picture. These photos are used to extract valuable data that can then be fed into the classification system for testing and training.

Immagulate et al. (2015) suggested using colour characteristics to analyse the skin illness psoriasis. Psoriasis comes in four different forms (guttate, nail, plaque, and pustular). Based on the characteristics of the colour histogram, the study's goal was to identify the various types of psoriasis for treatment. For the main feature extraction process, the RGB colour space image is converted to the HSV colour space. The H and S planes are then used to represent the colour histogram by dividing each plane into 11 bins, where each bin will indicate the number of colours. By combining the bins from the H and S plane, a total of 121 features are taken into account. The total number of pixels is then divided by the number of pixels in each bin to normalize these attributes.

### 5.3 System Design

Skin conditions are frequently difficult to identify at an early stage, and it is even more difficult to identify them independently. Melanoma is now widely recognized as the most dangerous skin cancer among all others because it is much more likely to spread to other bodily areas if not caught early and treated.

#### 5.3.1 Image Acquisition

In the context of image processing, the operation of obtaining a picture from a source—typically a hardware-based source—to communicate it via following a set of processes, can be broadly characterized. The workflow sequence for image processing always starts with the picture capture because processing an image is impossible without an image. The final image is unedited, which could be important in some industries where having a reliable starting point is essential. The input source functions within such precise and regulated conditions that it is possible to use the same image, if necessary, as the final product. This is one of the main objectives of this strategy, images nearly precisely duplicated under the same circumstances, making it simpler to identify and remove anomalous variables. Energy is reflected from the target via an optical system that concentrates, measures, and monitors the energy during the photo-taking procedure.

#### 5.3.2 Pre-Processing

When an image is acquired by a camera or similar imaging system, it is frequently not possible to use it directly with the visualization system for which it was built. Poor contrast, erratic intensity changes, or variations in illumination can all cause visual distortion, which must be corrected in the initial phases of image processing. The techniques for pre-processing images to get rid of these undesired traits and noise are covered in this section. The primary drawback of local averaging processes is their propensity to soften abrupt changes in intensity values in an image. A different strategy is to substitute the median of the grey values in the immediate area for each pixel value. This method of filtering is known as a Gaussian filter.

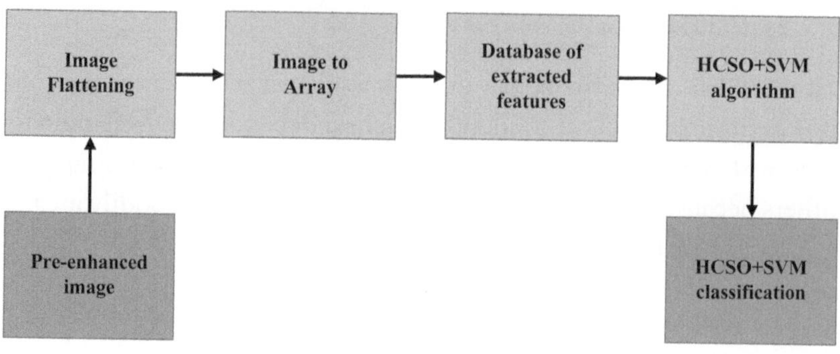


**Figure 5.4**　Pre-processing flow.

### 5.3.3 Image Pre-Processing

Images must first go through image pre-processing before being used for model training and inference. Alterations to the size, orientation, and colour are examples of this, but they are not the only changes that can be made (Ahmed et al., 2013). When there are multiple stages needed to prepare data for the user, this technique can be used at any initial or preliminary processing level. Figure 5.4 explains the pre-processing flow process in this proposed system.

### 5.3.4 Hybrid Cuckoo Search Optimization (HCSO)

For resolving mixed-variable engineering-design optimization issues, such as those involving integer, discrete, and continuous variables, and problem-specific constraints, a powerful cuckoo search and genetic algorithm hybrid (HCSO) is presented. The suggested method, HCSO, is then used to resolve three well-known design difficulties that have been documented in the literature (Sivanantham 2022). HCSO is applied first to 13 frequently used benchmark constrained optimization functions. Comparing the numerical findings from HCSO to other methods for solving problems involving restricted design optimization, they exhibit competitive performance. The proposed code's pseudo-HCSO method is shown in Figure 5.5.

### 5.3.5 Feature Extraction

The dimensionality reduction procedure, which divides the amount and complexity of an initial collection of raw data into manageable

**Begin**

Objective function f(x);

**Step 1: Initialization**. Randomize the population's start-up and set the generation counter to 1.

(Initialize each host nest containing an egg, which represents a potential answer to the stated issue, with the number of host nests being distributed at random);

**Step 2: Fitness evaluation.** Evaluate fitness f(x);

**While** (t< Max Generation) or (stop criterion); / **New population** /

Creating via genetic operators, a new population (selection, crossover and mutation)

Determine physical fitness (the best person can accomplish a Lévy flight)

Create a fresh idea (say, $x_{new}$) using Lévy flights;

Assess the product's fit and quality $Fx_{new}$;

Pick a random solution from $Np_{new}$ (let's say $x_j$) and assess its fitness ($F_j$);

**if**($Fx_{new}<F_j$) then

Change j to a different answer;

**end if**

Store the ideal remedy;

**t = t+1;**

**Step 3: End while**

**Step 4:** Find the top solution from the list of top solutions currently kept for each generation.

**End**

**Figure 5.5**  Pseudo code of proposed HCSO.

chunks, includes the feature extraction stage. As a result, processing will be simpler. The fact that these massive datasets contain a variety of distinctive elements is their most crucial feature. To process these variables, a lot of processing power is required. Feature extraction helps to find the best features in the enormous datasets to successfully reduce the amount of data by choosing and combining variables into features. These functions accurately and clearly represent the actual dataset while still being simple to use.

*5.3.5.1 Classifier as Support Vector Machines*  The machine learning paradigm known as the statistical learning theory forms the foundation of SVMs. To create the optimum separation borders across datasets, SVMs address a constrained quadratic optimization problem. However, additional kernel functions can be used to add various levels of flexibility and nonlinearity to the model, including linear, polynomial, radial basis functions, and sigmoid functions, but fundamental training procedures can only create linear separators, which is the idea behind an SVM.

One of the more well-known machine learning approaches, SVM can still be used to help with big data classification issues. In a big data setting, it might be especially helpful for multi-domain applications (Lingaraj et al., 2021). However, the SVM is computationally expensive and difficult mathematically. A machine learning approach that has skyrocketed in popularity for the analysis in recent years, SVMs uniquely provide balanced predicted performance, even in studies where sample sizes may be limited, because of their relative simplicity and flexibility in handling a range of classification challenges.

Compared to more traditional classifiers like decision trees and neural networks, SVMs provide a number of advantages. The fundamental goal of support vector training is to optimize a convex cost function. As a result, unlike back propagation neural networks, it eliminates the possibility of becoming stranded at local minima. Lowering the upper bound on the generalization error through the structural risk minimization (SRM) concept is the foundation of SVMs (Achakanalli & Sadashivappa 2014). As a result, SVMs are less likely to over fit than algorithms that apply the back propagation neural network's empirical risk minimization principle. Another benefit of SVMs is that, with the right kernel selection, they offer a unifying framework and it is possible to create learning machine designs like feed-forward neural networks and radial basis function (RBF) networks. The solitary binary classification output of SVMs has the limitation that no likelihood of class membership is offered.

In our study, image processing the Hybrid Cuckoo Search Optimization with Support Vector Machine algorithm (**HCSOSVM**) was used in addition to machine learning techniques to predict illnesses. To find these disorders, we used HCSO, SVM, and statistical analysis. The suggested application functions as a combination of medical treatment recommendations and detection. One of the more common issues in image processing is image classification. SVMs effectively analyse both structured and unstructured data, including text and images. Machine learning algorithms fall under the category of supervised learning models. SVM always needs clean data as an input.

The challenge in skin-disease identification is sorting the photos into many categories of skin illnesses.

## 5.4 Result and Discussion

Indian Health Service (IHS) recorded that more than 1 in every 10 persons in India will be impacted by skin ailments and 1 in every 100 persons will be severely ill with a skin disease. The suggested research system would serve as the first impetus for the development of an extensive strategy to test the general functioning and particular features on a variety of platform combinations. The methods are rigorously quality monitored. The technique uses modified, previously taught image recognizers to find photos of skin.

Four indexes Accuracy, Sensitivity, Specificity, and Time consumption are employed to evaluate the effectiveness of sentiment classification. The confusion matrix serves as the foundation for the general method of computing these indexes. Accuracy and error rate are two popular metrics for categorization performance. Accuracy is the ratio of correctly identified examples in all examples, whereas error rate uses incorrectly classified instances rather than successfully classified ones.

$$Accuracy = \frac{Tp + Tn}{Tp + Tn + Fp + Fn}$$

**TP (true positive):** The outcome of a forecast is positive and the true value is positive as well.

**TN (true negative):** A true negative outcome is one that should not appear negative yet does.

**FP (false positive):** A finding that suggests a certain condition is true even when it is false. However, it is referred to as a false positive if the true value is negative.

**FN (false negative):** When the outcome is projected to be negative, false negatives occur when the measured value is positive, but the result is positive.

*Compression result:* According to our suggested framework, many methods and algorithms may be used to forecast skin diseases.

*Accuracy:* A measurement or test's % accuracy is a gauge of how closely it resembles actual or ideal value. This ratio is the true value divided by the difference between the true and measured value.

$$Accuracy = \frac{(TP/TN)}{(TP + TN + FP + FN)}$$

Current technique yields an accuracy of 86.67 for detecting diseases using SVMs. Additionally, the artificial neural network's (ANN) output is more than 90.00. When compared to our suggested approach, which yields a superior result of 94.27, these two existing algorithms have somewhat worse results. Our proposed approach performs better in terms of accuracy when compared to the current system shown in Table 5.1.

According to Table 5.1, the results of the current algorithm are noted. To better comprehend the outcome of the current and suggested algorithms, the values in the table are plotted in the graph shown in Figure 5.6.

*Sensitivity:* The percentage of positive values out of all of the actual positive instances is known as sensitivity, recall, or the TP rate (TPR).

$$Sensitivity = \frac{TP}{TP + FN}$$

Numerous techniques and algorithms may be employed to forecast skin diseases in accordance with our proposed framework. Using SVMs, the present method detects diseases with a sensitivity of 86.67. The ANN's output is also more than 90.00. These two known methods perform somewhat worse than our proposed method, which achieves a better result of 94.27. When compared to the current system, our

**Table 5.1** Accuracy Table Containing Result Algorithm for Existing and Present System

| ALGORITHM | RESULT |
| --- | --- |
| SVM | 86.67 |
| ANN | 90.00 |
| HCSO+SVM | 94.27 |

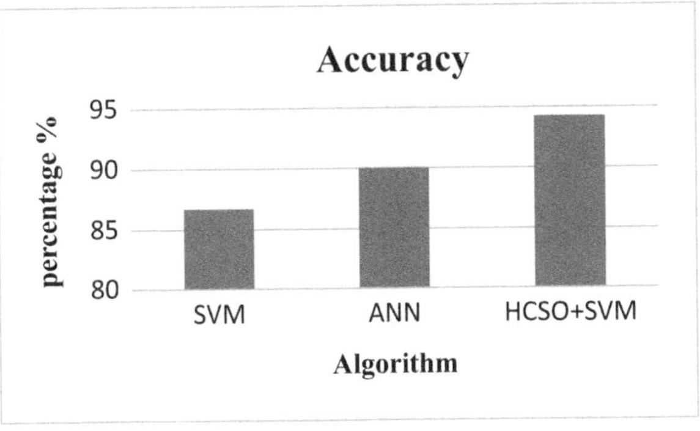


**Figure 5.6**   Graphical representation of the accuracy result.

proposed technique performs better in terms of sensitivity, as shown in Table 5.2.

The outcomes of the current algorithm are shown in Table 5.2. The values in the table are presented in Figure 5.7 to more clearly understand the results of the suggested and current algorithms.

*Specificity:* Calculating specificity involves taking the total number of correctly predicted negative outcomes and dividing that by the total number of negatives (SP (Specific Positive)), also known as the true negative rate (TNR). Specificity has a favourable value of 1.0, whereas the ideal value is 0.0.

$$\text{Specificity} = \frac{TN}{TN + FP}$$

According to our suggested framework, a variety of approaches and algorithms may be used to predict skin disorders. The current technique detects diseases with a specificity of 94.18 when using SVMs. The output of the ANN is likewise greater than 89.65. These two well-known techniques perform slightly worse than our suggested technique, which received a superior score of 84.25. Table 5.3

**Table 5.2**   Sensitivity Table Contains Result Algorithm for Existing and Present System

| ALGORITHM | RESULT |
|---|---|
| SVM | 88.38 |
| ANN | 90.56 |
| HCSO+SVM | 92.58 |

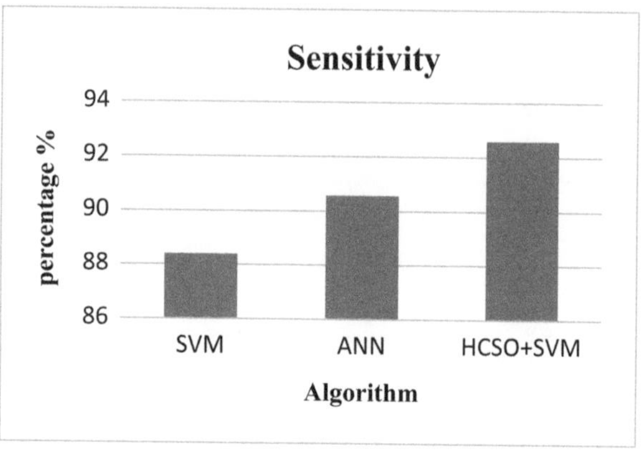

**Figure 5.7**   Graphical representation of the sensitivity result.

demonstrates how our suggested method outperforms the existing system in terms of specificity.

Table 5.3 displays the results of the present algorithm. To better comprehend the outcomes of the suggested and existing algorithms, the values from the table are shown in Figure 5.8.

***Time consumption (msec):*** According to our suggested framework, a variety of approaches and algorithms may be used to predict skin disorders. The current method detects diseases with a sensitivity of 31.25 using SVMs. The output of the ANN is likewise greater than 47.65. The prediction of diseases using the current algorithm has taken longer. According to our proposed technique, a person's skin illnesses can be discovered in as little as 24.14 seconds. Our suggested technique more efficiently uses time than the current system, as shown in Table 5.4.

Table 5.4 displays the results of the present algorithm. To better comprehend the outcomes of the suggested and existing algorithms, the values from the table are shown in Figure 5.9.

**Table 5.3**   Specificity Table Contains Result Algorithm for Present and Proposed System

| ALGORITHM | RESULT |
| --- | --- |
| SVM | 84.25 |
| ANN | 89.65 |
| HCSO+SVM | 94.18 |

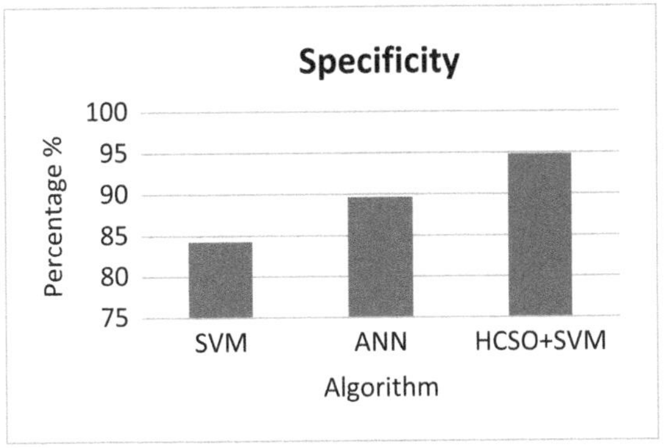


**Figure 5.8**  Graphical representation of the specificity result.

**Table 5.4**  Time Consumption Table Contains Result Algorithm for Present and Proposed System

| ALGORITHM | RESULT |
| --- | --- |
| SVM | 31.25 |
| ANN | 47.65 |
| HCSO+SVM | 24.14 |

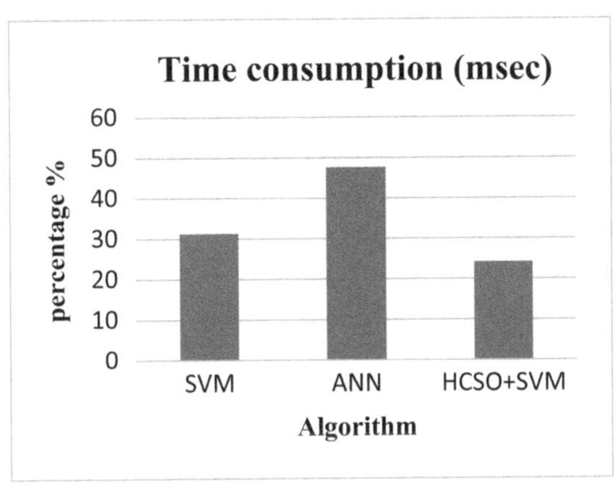


**Figure 5.9**  Graphical representation of time consumption.

## 5.5 Conclusion

In this study, a strategy for classifying dermoscopic pictures into melanoma and non-melanoma was proposed. Both colour and texture were utilized as feature types. Both Grey Level Co-occurrence Matrix (GLCM )and Local Binary Patterns (LBP) were used for texture characteristics. The categorization findings were more accurate when these features were combined. The suggested method increased the ability to categorize dermoscopic images into melanoma and non-melanoma groups. Experimentation was carried out on the dermIS standard dataset to assess the effectiveness and performance of the given model. Experiments yielded positive outcomes that support the suggested methodology. When paired with a substantial number of LBP features, GLCM can improve classification performance. The effectiveness of the system is measured using both qualitative and quantitative error measurements. Future work on this project will include SVM approaches, such as neural networks, for training classifiers based on a range of functions, polynomial functions, and radial basis functions. To determine whether a skin lesion is malignant, SVM classifier was applied to statistical texture features. By comparing each test set skin image to a training set skin image, the test set skin images were categorized.

# References


Achakanalli, Santosh, & Sadashivappa, G. (2014 May). Statistical Analysis of Skin Cancer Image –A Case Study, International Journal of Electronics and Communication Engineering (IJECE), 3(3), 1–10.

Ahmed, Kawsar, & Jesmin, Tasnuba (2013 January). Early Prevention and Detection of Skin Cancer Risk Using Data Mining, International Journal of Computer Applications, 62(4), 1–6.

Arivoli, P.V., Kaveri, E., & Chakravarthy, T. (2015). A survey on Segmentation and Classification Approach for Skin Medical Image. International Journal of Applied Engineering Research, 10(13), 33504–33509.

Barati, E., Saraee, M. H., Mohammadi, A., Adibi, N., & Ahmadzadeh, M. R. (2011). A Survey on Utilization of Data Mining Approaches for Dermatological (Skin) Diseases Prediction. Journal of Selected Areas in Health Informatics (JSHI), 2(3), 1–11.

Chaurasia, V., & Pal, S. (2019). Skin Diseases Prediction: Binary Classification Machine Learning and Multi Model Ensemble Techniques. Research Journal of Pharmacy and Technology, 12(8), 3829–3832.

Elngar, A. A., Kumar, R., Hayat, A., & Churi, P. (2021, August). Intelligent System for Skin Disease Prediction Using Machine Learning. Journal of Physics: Conference Series, 1998(1), 012037.

Immagulate, I., & Vijaya, M. S. (2015). Categorization of non-Melanoma Skin Lesion Diseases Using Support Vector Machine and Its Variants. International Journal of Medical Imaging, 3(2), 34–40.

Kanagaraj, G., Ponnambalam, S. G., Jawahar, N., & Nilakantan, J. M. (2014). An Effective Hybrid Cuckoo Search and Genetic Algorithm for Constrained Engineering Design Optimization. Engineering Optimization, 46(10), 1331–1351.

Kumar, Suresh, Kumar, Papendra, Gupta, Manoj, & Kumar, Ashok (2010). Performance Comparison of Median and Wiener Filter in Image De-noising. International Journal of Computer Application, 12(4), 27–31.

Lingaraj, M., Senthilkumar, A., & Ramkumar, J. (2021). Prediction of Melanoma Skin Cancer Using Veritable Support Vector Machine. Annals of the Romanian Society for Cell Biology, 25(4), 2623–2636.

Lu, Cheng, Mahmood, Muhammad, Jha, Naresh, & Manda, Mrinal (2013). Detection of Melanocytes in Skin Histopathological Images Using Radial Line Scanning. Journal of the Pattern Recognition, 46(2), 509–518.

Lu, Cheng, Mahmood, M., Jha, N., & Mandal, M. (2013). Automated Segmentation of the Melanocytes in Skin Histopathological Images. Journal of Biomedical and Health Informatics, IEEE, 17(2), 284–296.

Parikh, K. S., & Shah, T. P. (2016). Support Vector Machine–A Large Margin Classifier to Diagnose Skin Illnesses. Procedia Technology, 23, 369–375.

Patnaik, S. K., Sidhu, M. S., Gehlot, Y., Sharma, B., & Muthu, P. (2018). Automated Skin Disease Identification Using Deep Learning Algorithm. Biomedical & Pharmacology Journal, 11(3), 1429.

Porter, Robert S., Kasper, D. L., Braunwald, E., & Fauci, A. (2011). The Merck Manual', 'Harrison's Principles of Internal Medicine, 17th ed., McGraw-Hill, New York.

Sivanantham, K. (2022). Deep Learning-Based Convolutional Neural Network with Cuckoo Search Optimization for MRI Brain Tumour Segmentation. In Computational Intelligence Techniques for Green Smart Cities (pp. 149–168). Springer, Cham.

Srivastava, Chanchal, & Mishra, Saurabh Kumar et al. (Mar–Apr 2013). Performance Comparison of Various Filters and Wavelet Transform for Image De-Noising. IOSR Journal of Computer Engineering, 10(1), 55–63

Tajeripour, Farshad, Fekri-Ershad, Shervan, & Saberi, Mohammad (2012). An Innovative Skin Detection Approach Using Color Based Image Retrieval Technique. The International Journal of Multimedia & Its Applications (IJMA), 4(3).

Tymińska, Agata, Cichorek, Mirosława, Wachulska, Małgorzata, & Stasiewicz, Aneta, (2013). Skin Melanocytes: Biology and Development. Postepy dermatologii i alergologii, 30(1), 30–41.

Verma, A. K., Pal, S., & Kumar, S. (2019). Comparison of Skin Disease Prediction by Feature Selection Using Ensemble Data Mining Techniques. Informatics in Medicine Unlocked, 16, 100202.

# 6

# A Real-Time Detection of Eye Blinks from the Electroencephalogram

## A Morphological Component Analysis Approach

UDDIPAN HAZARIKA, BIDYUT BIKASH BORAH, SATYABRAT MALLA BUJAR BARUAH, AND SOUMIK ROY

### 6.1 Introduction

Recent scientific progress in industrialized nations has enabled the electroencephalogram (EEG) signal, sometimes known as a "brain signal", to be used for perceiving human emotions, brain activity, and other intellectual states of the human brain [1]. When addressing a traditional non-invasive interface for obtaining data about a person's mental state, EEG is often cited as the gold standard [2, 3]. EEG recordings from frontal channels are particularly susceptible to distortions caused by the subject's eye movements, making the detection and rejection of such aberrations a crucial step in improving the quality of EEG data. Eye blinks, cheek contraction/expansion, eye movement, etc., are common sources of artifacts in EEG readings. Artifacts in EEGs are often acquired from the frontal channels, and eye blinks are a major source of these artifacts. It is widely agreed that extracting the dynamics of eye blinking is a crucial step toward improving the quality of EEG data [4]. A positive deflection in the blinking mechanism is produced when the eyelid shuts, bringing the cornea closer to the site of the Fp1 electrode (left prefrontal lobe). The cornea moves away from Fp1 as the eyelid opens, resulting in a negative deflection [5].

Significant voltage peaks and minima in the EEG waveform are characteristic of eye blinks [6]. As a high-amplitude artifact signal, blinking is especially troubling for EEG analysis. However, artifacts of this type may be used as trigger factors for various controlling applications, such as Internet of Things (IoT)-based Brain Computer interface devices used



DOI: 10.1201/9781032667508-6

for controlling arm movement, wheelchair movements, home automation, etc. [7, 8]. In the literature [9], a mean threshold approach was suggested to identify eye blinking from electroencephalography based on blinking or an opened eye. The literature [10] also suggests that a common technique for removing eye-blink artifacts uses adaptive noise cancellation (ANC) and discrete wavelet transform (DWT) methods. Given that the eye blink is an peripheral trigger artifact with a higher extent of association and correspondence with frontal EEG channels than other artifact-generating causes due to its location closer to the Fp1 channel electrode and significant amplitude, the literature [11] proposes an independent component analysis (ICA) method based on correlation or the extent of similarity and the feature of power spreading over the EEG frequency range to automatically detect an eye-blink entity.

The proposed study introduces a Morphological Component Analysis (MCA)-based real-time approach for detecting blinks from EEG signals collected using a TGAM EEG sensor. Basis matrices are sparse representations of signals like eye blinks and EEGs, and they may be quickly and effectively generated with the help of Short-Time Fourier Transform (STFT). The main benefit of the real-time computing of basis matrices is the reduced need for memory. The work is divided into many parts depending on the following sections: EEG collection, preprocessing of EEG data, MCA, findings demonstrating eye blinking extraction, discussions, and conclusion.

## 6.2 Methods

The methods of the proposed framework mainly flow in an ascending order from: acquisition of the raw EEG data from the subject; processing of the acquired signals, including design of a band pass filter and a notch filter; then segmenting the cleaned signals; MCA for breaking down the signals into distinct components; and finally extracting/detecting eye blinks from the EEG signal.

### 6.2.1 Acquisition of EEG Biosignal

The proposed system employs the NeuroSky TGAM module [12, 13] for biosignal acquisition and processing. The Think Gear ASIC module serves as the foundation for the programmable TGAM module,

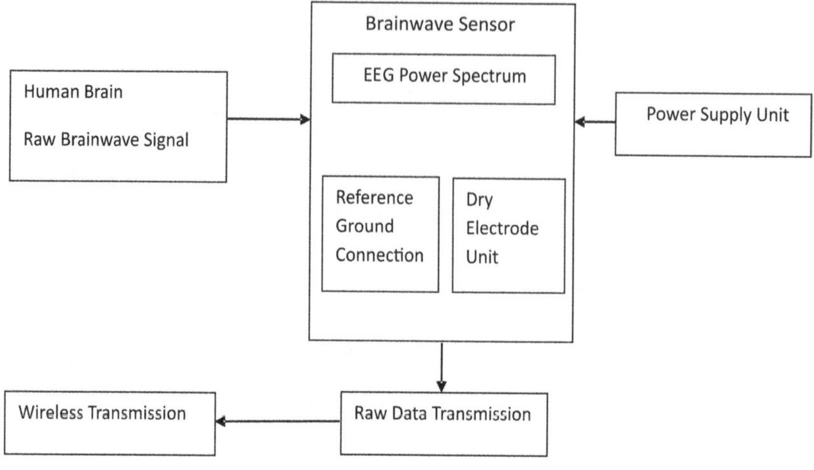


**Figure 6.1** Functioning basis diagram of the electroencephalogram acquiring arrangement.

which has a sampling frequency of 512 Hz. The module includes an integrated filtering and de-noising circuit that can automatically remove different types of noises. The NeuroSky TGAM module consists of an electrode as the reference point on the A1 position or the ear clip and an EEG biopotential measuring electrode that is placed in the Fp1 location on the forehead above the eye. The electrodes are dry electrodes; therefore, no skin readiness or conductive pastes are necessary. The diagrammatic representation of the EEG biosignal collection system is shown in Figure 6.1. Coupling the TGAM module to a Bluetooth module allows the latter to send packets containing EEG data to the processing block via a unidirectional communication link.

### 6.2.2 Brain Signal Processing

A third-order median filter was utilized to initially eliminate noise from the raw EEG data. Following the first filtering of the signals, a composite of both a low-pass filter and a high-pass filter was employed to further enhance their quality and refinement. These filters were created using a 5th-order Butterworth filter with 50 Hz and 0.5 Hz cutoff frequencies, respectively, for the low- and high-pass filtration. The Butterworth filter, used in signal processing, has a pass band frequency response that is as flat as feasible.

Subsequently, a notch filter was employed to eradicate the interference caused by the AC powerline. Signals were also de-noised using a multi-layer wavelet decomposition based de-noising approach. There were a total of five wavelet layers, with Symlets as the "mother" wavelet. The Savitzky-Golay filter was then used to the signals to smooth them out.

The obtained time series signals were filtered and then segmented using a sliding window in time domain. The procedure entailed the subsequent stages. At first, a window with a width of 4 seconds was employed to iterate through the time-domain information. The window width was selected on basis of the literature [14–16]. The proposed method began with a 50% overlapping window.

Afterward, several values for the width of the sliding window and the overlapping window were tested until the best level of accuracy was attained with a sliding window of 4 seconds and an overlying window of 3 seconds. The chops of the time-domain biosignal were subsequently transformed to the frequency domain using the Fast Fourier Transformation technique. The wavelet transformation process was employed to decompose the segmented signals to the time-frequency domain. A 4-second sliding window with an overlap of 3 seconds was used in the proposed model. Due to the blinking dynamics and time duration of the blinking signals, the overlap window was selected as 3 seconds. If the window was considered to be very small or moderate, then there is a high probability of blinking signal loss.

### 6.2.3 Analysis of The Morphological Components of EEG Signals

MCA is a technique for breaking down a signal into its individual components. The approach permits reconstruction using a sparse representation based on the assumption that each signal constituent has its own unique morphology [17, 18].

Suppose an EEG signal $x$ has $P$ number of its unique components $x_1, x_2, ..., x_P$ depicting the useful information of the brain state as well as the noise contaminations, and every unique apparatus is signified sparsely using the basis notations as $\psi_1, \psi_2, ..., \psi_P$, respectively. Now, the brain signal $x$ can be denoted with the help of the basis notations as written in Eq. (6.1).

$$x = \psi_1\mu_1 + \psi_2\mu_2 + \cdots + \psi_P\mu_P \tag{6.1}$$

The notations $\mu_1$, $\mu_2$,.., $\mu_P$ as written in Eq. (6.1) are the projection coefficients of the EEG signal's unique components $x_1, x_2, ..., x_P$ on the basis pursuit $\psi_1, \psi_2, ..., \psi_P$ and $P$ is the total number of significant biosignal components. In this particular framework, the two primary constituents of the brain signal $x$ are considered as $x_1$ and $x_2$ (So, $P = 2$).

In this particular approach, $x$, $x_1$, and $x_2$ are considered as the original EEG signal collected with the help of the TGAM module, filtered EEG, and eye-blink artifact signal correspondingly depending on the ADC values. The two primary component signals namely $x_1$ and $x_2$ can be depicted as linear combination of the bases $\psi_1$ and $\psi_2$, respectively. To satisfy the assumption of MCA, it is crucial to have a dictionary of bases $\psi_1$ and $\psi_2$ such that for each signal component in $x$ i.e., $x_1$ and $x_2$ is sparse in either $\psi_1$, or sparse in $\psi_2$ [14].

By finding out the coefficients $\mu_1$ and $\mu_2$ from Eq. (6.1), the concerned biosignal $x$ can then be decomposed using MCA as written in Eq. (6.2).

$$x = {\psi_1}^T \mu_1 + {\psi_2}^T \mu_2 = x_1 + x_2 \tag{6.2}$$

By employing the basis pursuit strategy, the coefficients $\mu_1$ and $\mu_2$ in Eq. (6.2) may be determined by $l_1$-norm minimization [19].

### 6.2.4 MCA-Based Distinction of Eye-Blink Artifacts from EEG

The brain signal exhibits non-stationarity, with a gradual variation in its spectral information over time, rendering it appropriate for analysis using STFT. A mathematical interpretation of the STFT of a signal $x[n]$ is depicted in Eq. (6.3).

$$STFT\left\{x[n]\right\} = \sum_{n=0}^{L+1}\left\{x[n-k]w[n]\right\}e^{-jwn} \tag{6.3}$$

The sliding window, denoted as $\omega[n]$, highlights local frequency components inside it. The length both of the window is represented by $L$. A longer window length offers more frequency resolution, while a shorter window length gives higher temporal resolution. The technique depicted in Figure 6.2 was utilized to achieve real-time blink segregation from the original brain signal.

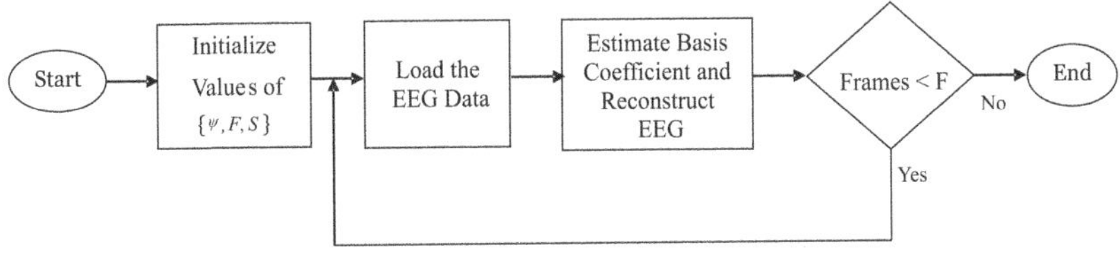

**Figure 6.2**  Blinking extraction flowchart from EEG.

Initially, the parameters were initialized, including the basis matrices $\psi = (\psi_1, \psi_2)$, the maximum number of frames ($F$), and the total amount of samples per frame ($S$). The basis matrices for the EEG and blinking artifacts were calculated by utilizing STFT. A wide window length ($\approx 2S$) was used for the EEG signal, while a shorter window length of around *500 ms* was used for the identification of the eye blinks. This choice was made since most eye blinks had a duration between *200* and *400 ms*. The basis coefficients were determined repeatedly using a basis pursuit method. Subsequently, the cleaned EEG signal was reconstructed using the acquired coefficients.

## 6.3  Results and Discussions

The proposed framework compared the raw EEG signal acquired as detailed in Section 2.1 with the cleaned EEG signal seen in Figure 6.3 to determine how well this approach performed. A pair of highly correlated signals has a correlation coefficient of 1, and the correlation coefficient of an uncorrelated signal pair gives a value of 0. It is essential to note that even if the algorithm is excellent, if the acquired EEG comprises numerous eye blinks, it will not correlate with the purified brain signal. This is despite the fact that this method is widely used as a comparison measure of signal similarity. More than 60 frames of EEG information were acquired and using a 4-second window with an overlap of 3 seconds, processed in real time to evaluate the approach provided in this study for detecting eye blinks.

Figure 6.4 demonstrates that when the subject's eyelid shuts, the cornea moves towards the Fp1 electrode and generates a crest with a positive deviation. Similarly, as the eyelid opens, the cornea moves apart from the left frontal pole and produces a trough with a negative deviation.

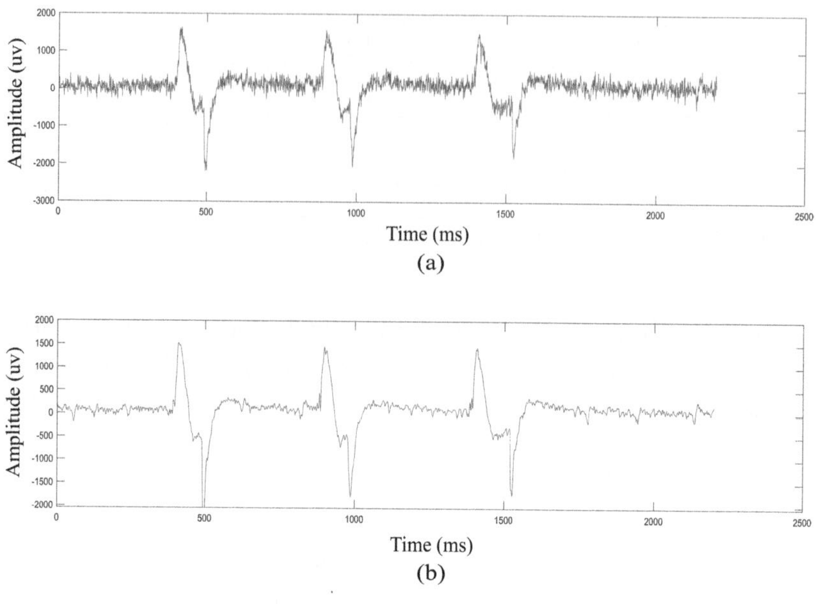

**Figure 6.3** (a) A raw brain signal extracted from the subject using TGAM and (b) a filtered EEG signal.

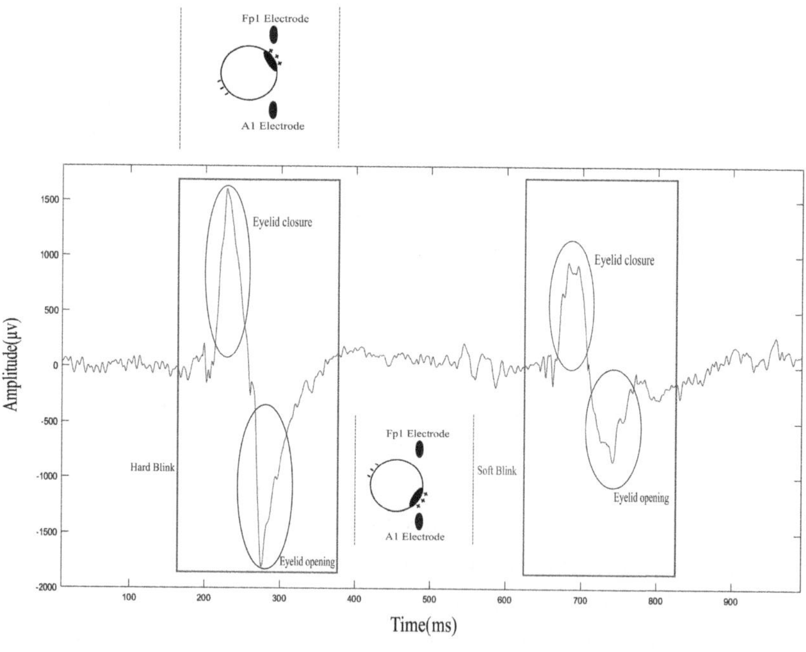



**Figure 6.4** Graphical representation of the extracted soft blinks and hard blinks.

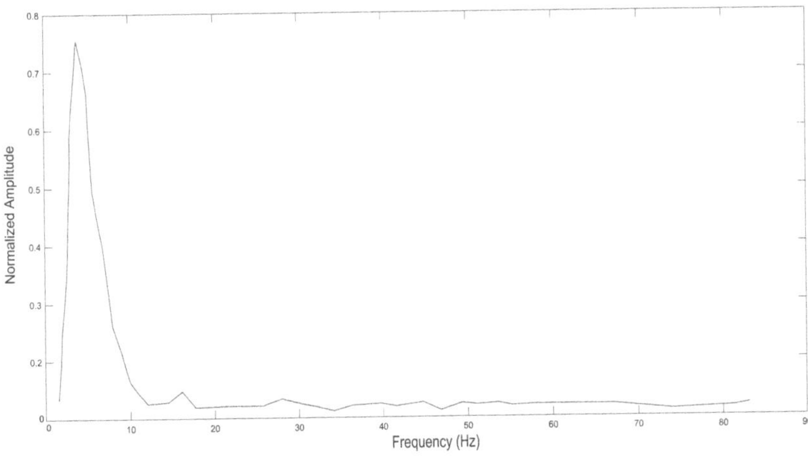

**Figure 6.5**  Graphical representation of the frequency response of eye blink signal.

As illustrated in Figure 6.5, the eye-blinking signal has a very low frequency range of 0–13 Hz. The correlation coefficient between the unprocessed EEG and the processed signal ranged from 0.75 to 0.94, with the exact value dependent on the extent of contamination caused by eye blinks. As the number of eye blinks increases and contamination worsens, the correlation coefficient approaches a value that is decreasing. Table 6.1 shows the numerical estimation of two performance criteria, namely, correlation coefficient and execution time per frame upon testing the algorithm on different EEG datasets, namely, SEED dataset [20, 21] and SEED-IV datasets [22], considering particularly the Fp1 channel neural dynamics.

In terms of execution time per frame and correlation coefficients, Figure 6.6 provides a head-to-head comparison of the performance of the SEED-IV and SEED datasets. The EEGs of 15 subjects were recorded for both the SEED and SEED-IV databases. As can be seen in the bar graph, the execution time per frame rises when the correlation coefficient is low, i.e., in between (0.75–0.84), because these

**Table 6.1**  Performance Evaluation Chart of the Proposed Algorithm

| | PERFORMANCE EVALUATION CHART | |
|---|---|---|
| SL. NO | PERFORMANCE CRITERIA | VALUES |
| 1 | Correlation coefficient (highly contaminated by eye-blink signals) | 0.75 to 0.84 |
| 2 | Correlation coefficient (less contaminated by eye-blink signals) | 0.84 to 0.94 |
| 3 | Average execution time per frame | 27 msec |

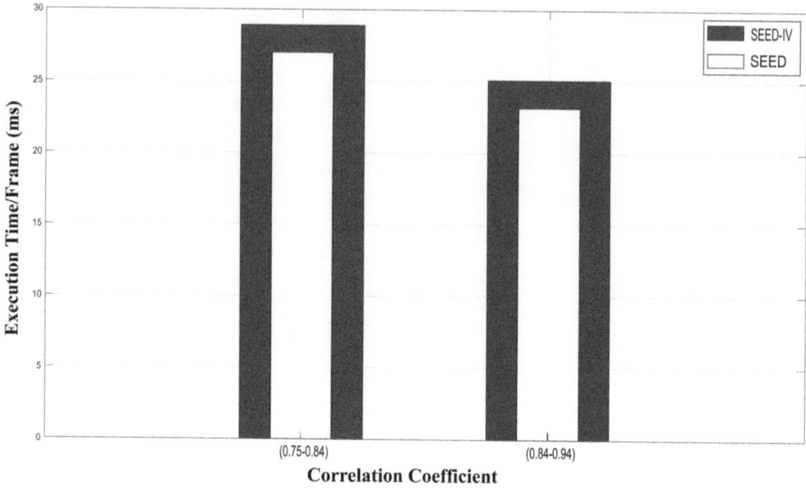


**Figure 6.6** Comparison of performance criteria between the SEED-IV and SEED datasets.

signals are heavily contaminated with blink artifacts. As the correlation coefficient between the unfiltered EEG data and blink artifacts-free signal increases, i.e., in between (0.84–0.94), the execution time per frame decreases as these signals are less contaminated with eye-blink artifacts.

## 6.4 Conclusion

This research framework proposes the use of a morphological learning-based system to automate the process of extracting out the artifact of eye blinking in real-time from EEG recordings in the Fp1 channel. The MCA algorithm has been found to be effective even when dealing with EEG data that has been tainted by eye blinks. The proposed algorithm was evaluated on the SEED and SEED-IV datasets, where it was found that there is a significant correlation between the raw brain signal and the purified signal after the eye blinks have been detected, and that the coefficient of correlation tends to decrease as the contamination of eye blinks in a particular EEG recording increases. The findings demonstrate that MCA has the ability to effectively distinguish eye blinks from the unprocessed brain state information in real-time. Despite being a looping technique, the mean duration for sweeping one frame (512 samples) of the acquired EEG using MCA was *28.9 milliseconds*, with a standard variation of *0.10 milliseconds*. This was achieved on a desktop PC equipped with a 64-bit operating system and a 2.90 GHz CPU. The existing architecture could be expanded in the future to create a system that can detect and extract artifacts such as cardiac activity, muscle activity, cheek movement, and so on. The capacity to identify eye blinks can be integrated with other occurrences, such as motor imagery in neuro-feedback, control applications in neuro-rehabilitation, application control through brain-computer interface, and IoT-enabled devices.

### Acknowledgement

The first author acknowledges the Department of Science and Technology, Government of India for supporting this research work financially under DST-INSPIRE Fellowship Scheme. INSPIRE-Fellow Registration Number: [IF210446].

# References


1. Kumar, J. Satheesh and P. Bhuvaneswari. "Analysis of electroencephalography (EEG) signals and its categorization—a study." Procedia Engineering 38 (2012): 2525–2536.
2. Pushpa, S., S. CN and P. G. Student. "EEG based brain-computer interface for controlling home appliances." International Journal of Innovative Research in Science, Engineering and Technology 3297.6 (2007): 9870–9877.
3. Sanei, Saeid and Jonathon A. Chambers. EEG Signal Processing. John Wiley & Sons, 2013.
4. Chang, Won-Du, et al. "Detection of eye blink artifacts from single prefrontal channel electroencephalogram." Computer Methods and Programs in Biomedicine 124 (2016): 19–30.
5. Abo-Zahhad, Mohammed, Sabah M. Ahmed and Sherif N. Abbas. "A new multi-level approach to EEG based human authentication using eye blinking." Pattern Recognition Letters 82 (2016): 216–225.
6. b Abd Rani, Mohd Shaifulrizal. "Detection of eye blinks from EEG signals for home lighting system activation." 2009 6th International Symposium on Mechatronics and its Applications. IEEE, 2009.
7. Rihana, S., P. Damien and T. Moujaess. "EEG-eye blink detection system for brain computer interface." Converging Clinical and Engineering Research on Neurorehabilitation. Springer, Berlin, Heidelberg, 2013. 603–608.

8. Varela, Michael. "Raw EEG signal processing for BCI control based on voluntary eye blinks." 2015 IEEE Thirty Fifth Central American and Panama Convention (CONCAPAN XXXV). IEEE, 2015.

9. Nguyen, T., et al. "A mean threshold algorithm for human eye blinking detection using EEG." 4th International Conference on Biomedical Engineering in Vietnam. Springer, Berlin, Heidelberg, 2013.

10. Ghosh, Rajdeep, Nidul Sinha and Saroj Kumar Biswas. "Automated eye blink artefact removal from eeg using support vector machine and autoencoder." IET Signal Processing 13.2 (2019): 141–148.

11. Kong, Wanzeng, et al. "Automatic and direct identification of blink components from scalp EEG." Sensors 13.8 (2013): 10783–10801.

12. Yin, Liyong, Chao Zhang and Zhijie Cui. "Experimental research on realtime acquisition and monitoring of wearable EEG based on TGAM module." Computer Communications 151 (2020): 76–85.

13. Zhang, Lu, Qingsong Lv and Yishen Xu. "Single channel brain-computer interface control system based on TGAM module." 2017 10th International Congress on Image and Signal Processing, BioMedical Engineering and Informatics (CISPBMEI). IEEE, 2017.

14. Bobin, Jérôme, et al. "Morphological component analysis: An adaptive thresholding strategy." IEEE Transactions on Image Processing 16.11 (2007): 2675–2681.

15. Nguyen, Hien M., Jingyuan Chen and Gary Glover. "Morphological component analysis of functional MRI brain networks." IEEE Transactions on Biomedical Engineering 69.10 (2022): 3193–3204.

16. Starck, Jean-Luc, D. L. Donoho and Michael Elad. Redundant multiscale transforms and their application for morphological component separation. No. DAPNIA-2004-88. CM-P00052061, 2004.

17. Nisar, Shibli, Omar Usman Khan and Muhammad Tariq. "An efficient adaptive window size selection method for improving spectrogram visualization." Computational Intelligence and Neuroscience 2016 (2016): 13.

18. Starck, J-L., et al. "Morphological component analysis." Wavelets XI. Vol. 5914. SPIE, 2005.

19. Selesnick, Ivan W. "Sparse signal representations using the tunable Q-factor wavelet transform." Wavelets and Sparsity XIV. Vol. 8138. SPIE, 2011.

20. Duan, Ruo-Nan, Jia-Yi Zhu and Bao-Liang Lu. "Differential entropy feature for EEG-based emotion classification." 2013 6th International IEEE/EMBS Conference on Neural Engineering (NER). IEEE, 2013.

21. Zheng, Wei-Long and Bao-Liang Lu. "Investigating critical frequency bands and channels for EEG-based emotion recognition with deep neural networks." IEEE Transactions on Autonomous Mental Development 7.3 (2015): 162–175.

22. Zheng, Wei-Long, et al. "Emotionmeter: A multimodal framework for recognizing human emotions." IEEE Transactions on Cybernetics 49.3 (2018): 1110–1122.

7

# Application of Machine Learning for Prediction of Anxiety and Depression among Elderly Patients

## A Critical Review and Analysis

### GAYATRI PANDA

## 7.1 Introduction

In this fast-paced world and with more involvement required in the workplace by their adult children, the elderly are more prone to mental disorders. Anxiety and depression are the two common mental disorders that have expanded into elderly life. Gerard and Nancy (2010) in their study elaborated that depression lead to cognitive disabilities and also that depression had a bidirectional relationship with obesity. Treating anxiety and depression disorders among elderly patients will enhance their quality of life and develop better social activities and cognitive abilities (Saraçli et al., 2015). Islam et al. (2018) stated that social media network usage provided an opportunity to share emotions, pictures, and feelings which provided a way to release the level of anxiety among elderly people and minimize the level of health-associated risk and disorders. Mohr et al. (2017) discussed the important point that sensors and personal gadgets are considered important tools for analyzing personal life and understanding human behavior, feelings, and sentiments. Shinde and Rajeswari (2018) opined that machine-learning operations will enable one to understand the health risks and predict the information for taking precautionary steps for better results. Andrews (2018) attempted to develop a model for the early identification of anxiety and depression disorders among elderly patients using machine learning and suggested

DOI: 10.1201/9781032667508-7

**99**

that identification in the early stage and with the help of interview sessions would result in minimizing the disorders and developing stability among patients.

Hatton et al. (2019) explained the application of machine learning helps in the persistent diagnosis of anxiety and depression symptoms among elderly patients. Kumar et al. (2020) and Pandit et al. (2023) focused on studying the prediction of the severity level of anxiety and depression symptoms, and it was observed that the use of a hybrid algorithm provided better results compared to a single algorithm. Nemesure et al. (2021) explored the relevance of adequate living conditions and maintaining health insurance as having a close connection with depressive disorders; these two conditions could affect whether the patient was relaxed and able to overcome deficiencies. Identifying important predictors can enable the detection of disorders at a faster pace and can help suggest treatment measures. On the other hand, machine learning algorithms provide excellent results in predicting clinically significant aspects.

There is a paucity of existing studies on anxiety and depression disorders among elderly patients, which is of paramount importance and considered one of the primary research gaps by researchers (Kunze et al., 2021; van Eeden et al., 2021). This prompted the researcher to explore this area. Thus, the present study is a unique approach to understanding the present research state of the condition through a "systematic literature review and bibliometric analysis" for predicting anxiety and depression among elderly patients using machine learning. To justify the stated research gap, the following questions have been framed by the researcher:

Q1. What role does machine learning play in predicting anxiety and depression disorders among elderly patients?

Q2: Mention the significant journals and countries with profound publications on this topic.

Q3: Mention the noteworthy authors and the co-authorship trend.

Q4: Elucidate keyword statistics and mentioned articles and develop topic mapping on this area.

Q5: Explain the forthcoming thematic areas of machine learning in predicting anxiety and depression disorders among elderly patients.

Based on the comprehensive discussion, the resulting questions and objectives have been developed:

- "To evaluate research studies on the application of machine learning in predicting anxiety and depression among elderly patients."
- "To formulate the research streams in machine learning in predicting anxiety and depression among elderly patients."
- "To develop a framework for upcoming researchers to understand the application of machine learning in predicting disorders among elderly patients."

The current study adopted a systematic review approach to machine learning applications in predicting anxiety and depression disorders among elderly patients and focused on achieving the framed objectives. The research work attempts to analyze the existing articles on the application of machine learning in anxiety and depression disorders among elderly patients to measure the current state of research studies. The current study points attention toward understanding the contribution in terms of various contributors, countries, and yearly trends as well as bibliometric and network analysis.

This chapter contains in seven sections. The first section was discussed in the introduction, which enabled the researcher to frame the stated question and objectives. Section 7.2 discusses a background analysis of articles and Section 7.3 discusses the study's procedure, which covers the database, keywords, and article selection. Section 7.4 explains bibliometric, network analysis, and developing research streams on machine learning in predicting anxiety and depression among elderly patients. Section 7.5 describes the implications of the study. Section 7.6 explains the research discussion and Section 7.7 elaborates on the conclusion of the study.

## 7.2 Current Literature Analysis

Literature analysis is an imperative mechanism that helps to understand, map, and measure the present literature to highlight the boundaries of information and identify possible gaps (Tranfield et al., 2003). The researcher considered the systematic literature review because, unlike traditional reviews, the systematic literature review uses article collection methods that are replicable, exact, and free from presumptions on the significance of the selected literature (Pickering & Byrne, 2014).

In the changing social, technological, and environmental conditions, people face more changes and challenges. Elderly patients need to understand various aspects to cope with societal conditions. Islam et al. (2018) expressed their concern about understanding the relevance of social network platforms for developing significant moods and attitudes among elderly people. It was identified that the decision tree technique of machine learning can provide highly efficient solutions to manage depressive disorders. Wang et al. (2019) explored the relevance of the street environment. It is signified that older people consider their neighborhood as an important predictor of their perception. Perceived perception can extend their anxiety and depression symptoms; thus, machine learning could assess different attributes and a significant outcome could create a check for better results. Su et al. (2021) and Bhatnagar et al. (2023) suggested the decision-support system approach developed in predictive models through machine learning techniques can be valuable for doctors and medical practitioners for the early detection of disorders. Following that research, Rajawat et al. (2021) discussed that fusion-based developed models such as the use of robots in the form of social animals and humanoids can detect depression symptoms among elderly patients and aid in the development of better treatment measures. Ali and Azhar (2022) explained machine learning algorithms such as logistic regression can be used to predict disorders among elderly patients.

Mental stability is one of the most important aspects specifically among elderly people. The measures to introduce machine learning in the health sector became a significant parameter to expand the scope of new treatment opportunities in this area. Considering the existing review of studies, the researcher recognized the following gaps such as (1) The exploration of machine learning in the health sector with specific relation to predicting anxiety and depression disorders among elderly patients is very scarce (Priya et al., 2020); and (2) The existing studies have accelerated various aspects on the application of machine learning, but no study has developed any future research framework for upcoming researchers (Nemesure et al., 2021). Hence, from the identified gaps, there is a great need to explore the integration of machine learning in the prediction of mental disorders among elderly patients, which stimulates the design of the current study.

## 7.3 Study Procedure

The research work aims to understand, analyze, and examine the existing literature studies on machine learning applications for predicting anxiety and depression disorders. The research attempts to understand the role of machine learning in diagnosing anxiety and depression from health-related factors. The rationality behind adopting the technique enables us to understand to what extent the technique enhances the ability to identify mental disorders among elderly patients, provide necessary information to health practitioners, and provide a solution to overcome the conditions. However, mixture studies were developed on an array of themes related to machine learning applications. Nevertheless, only limited studies have discussed simple linear regression (SLR) and bibliometric analysis of studies on machine learning applications in predicting anxiety and depression disorders among elderly people. The research adopted a sequential approach to justify the stated questions and objectives.

The current research work aims to develop and present the extracted articles based on citation, co-citation, and cluster basis as well as understand the future viewpoints to justify the stated questions. The study mostly measures the present and future trends in machine learning applications in predicting mental disorders. Lastly, the most imperative reason for the present study is machine learning needs to be endorsed in the field of health sciences in a broader way, which inspired the researcher to progress with an amalgamated work that can be a value-addition to the area. Therefore, the current study is considered as one value-added research work for health practitioners, providing a tangible idea for their impending research endeavor. Figure 7.1 explains the flow chart and study procedure for article extraction.

### 7.3.1 Selection of Repository

The current study decided on the Scopus repository for extracting the articles because it is considered one of the most robust repository by

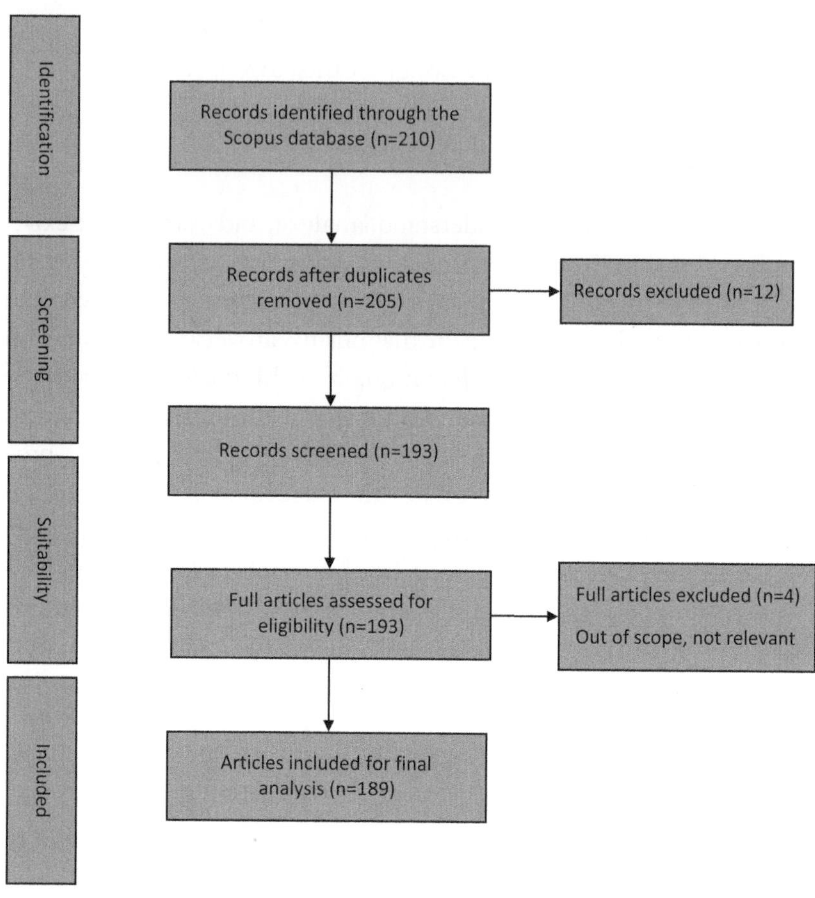


**Figure 7.1**   Flowchart for article extraction.

researchers for extracting literature (Meester et al., 2017; Montoya et al., 2018) for bibliometric data. Thus, the research work used the Scopus repository to collect the data and to cover a broad range of literature, and the study outlined a blend of keywords elaborated upon in the subsequent sections.

### 7.3.2  *Selecting Keywords*

The study adopted an SLR of articles on machine learning in predicting anxiety and depression disorder (Trevisani & Tuzzi 2015). The prime concern while classifying articles is the range of keywords. Thus, the acknowledged keywords were considered in this current study to accumulate studies on machine learning applications in predicting anxiety and depression disorders among elderly patients.

*"Machine learning" OR "ML" AND "Anxiety" AND" Depression" AND "Elderly" OR "Aged patients"*

### 7.3.3  Cleaning of Articles

The study followed exclusion/inclusion criteria to identify the required articles from the Scopus database. After extracting a total of 210 articles, the researcher adopted the following inclusion criteria, which led to finding the appropriate number of articles to be considered for further analysis by considering: the document type, "article, conference, book chapter," in relation to article type; "Journal, conference proceedings"; language, "English"; and, lastly, keyword type, "Exact keywords" such as "Machine learning," "ML" "anxiety," "depression," "Elderly", "Aged patients." This resulted into the abstraction of 189 documents.

### 7.3.4  Assembling Articles

The study acknowledged the 189 documents for developing the present work. The CSV (comma-separated values) format document extracted from the Scopus database was taken for bibliometric analysis. The researcher verified systematically the concept of "machine learning," "anxiety," and "depression" in the title as well as in abstract respectively.

## 7.4  Analysis and Findings

### 7.4.1  Source-wise Statistics

The next section discusses the results and findings of the study by identifying the sources with the maximum publication, as well as providing information on yearly trends, country-wise publication, prolific authors as well as information on network analysis based on author/co-authorship, keyword statistics, citation, and co-citations. The prime objective is to assemble the existing work and develop a plan

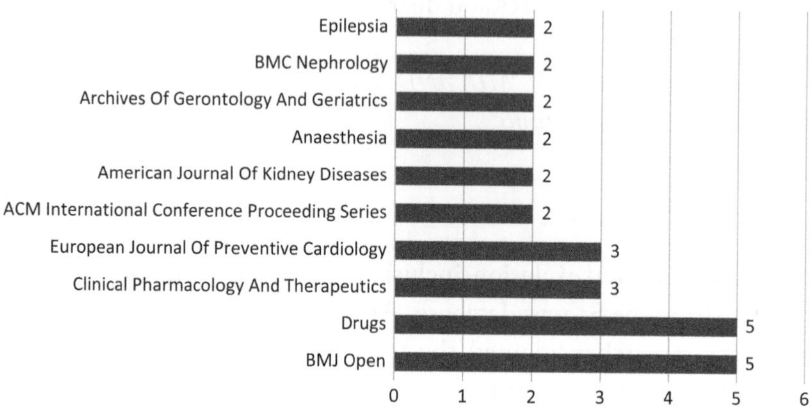



**Figure 7.2** Sourcewise statistics.

for future researchers in machine learning applications in predicting anxiety and depression disorders among elderly patients.

Figure 7.2 shows the publication trend of journals. The considered 189 papers in the study are published in 156 journals out of which the top ten journals were considered. The top journal belongs to the British Medical Association, which has five papers to its credit, whereas the remaining papers appear in other leading publications. However, the present set of articles are still few, which improves the scope and provides transparent ways for other researchers to investigate the area and supply more pertinent studies.

### 7.4.2 Publication Trend

Figure 7.3 shows the publication trend on a yearly basis. It suggests that there was significant growth in publications from the year 2018 and indicates that the researchers are consistently working to develop research studies in the area and focusing on studies that will add value to the existing research state. With new research comes new models, strategies, and measures to predict the mental disorders among elderly patients, providing solutions to manage the state of disorder and lead a healthy and stable life. The progressive trend denotes a wider scope in the research topic and upcoming researchers should develop studies for better results.

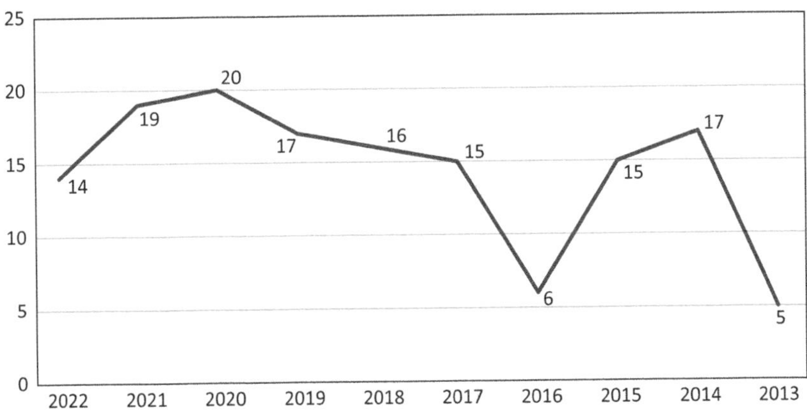



**Figure 7.3** Publication trend.

### 7.4.3 Country Statistics

Figure 7.4 presents the country statistics, which shows the countries based on two criteria: developed or developing nations. The developing countries consist of China and the developed countries include Australia, South Korea, Spain, France, Germany, Canada, Italy, United Kingdom, United States. The identified top ten countries are developed nations. The United States is at the top position with maximum publication of 55 articles, whereas Australia has least publications. However, it indicates there is huge scope for every country to

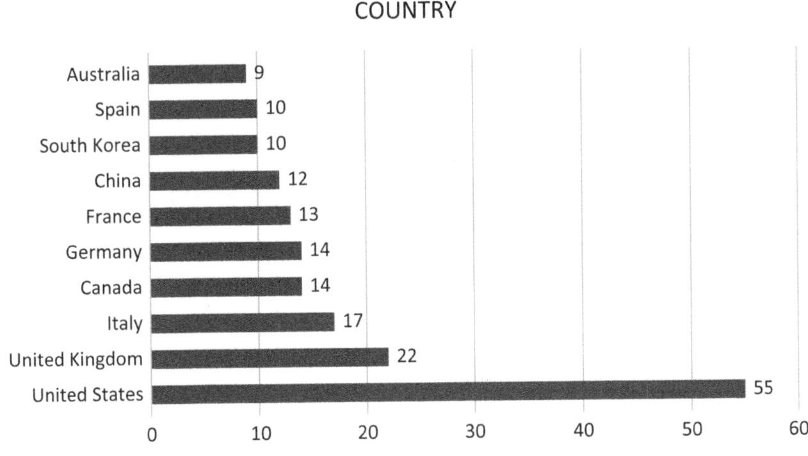



**Figure 7.4** Country statistics.

develop research studies and contribute to the existing research state with new predictive models, measures, and solutions for predicting and treating mental disorders among elderly patients.

### 7.4.4 Network Analysis on Author/Co-authorship

The next sections discuss network analysis maps on identifying the relationship between existing authors and co-authors and identifications of highly cited articles based on citation and co-citation analysis, measuring the keyword statistics. A co-authorship network map reveals the relationship between authors and provides scope to develop broader social networks (Kumar, 2015). The developed map indicates the author/co-authorship relationship. The study included an inclusion criterion to identify the significant contributor; from a total of 1128 authors, only the authors who have collaborated in two research papers and have at least one citation have been included. Figure 7.5 demonstrates the author and co-authorship map. Finally, it led to the identification of 20 authors who have collaborated and worked in the area of machine learning for predicting anxiety and depression disorder among elderly patients. Thus, the researcher can conclude

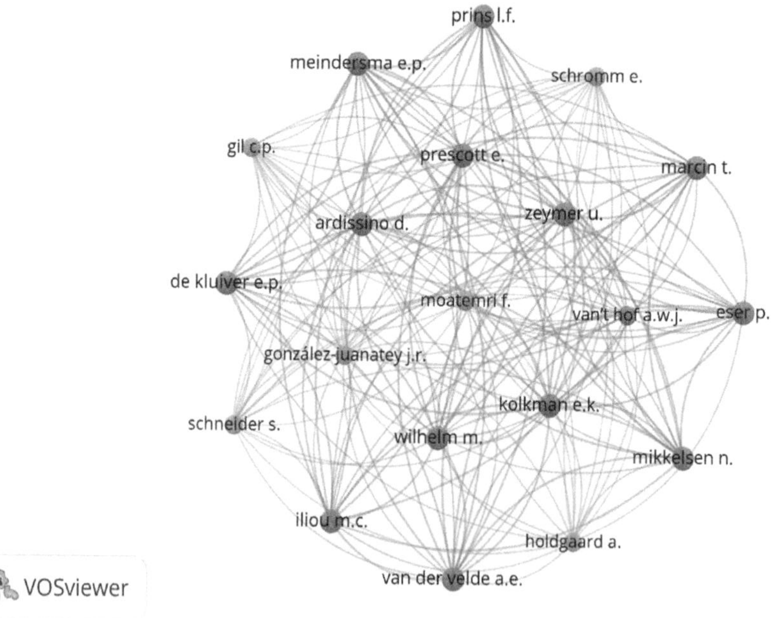


**Figure 7.5**   Author/co-authorship.

that very few authors have collaborated and created research studies, which leaves an opportunity for future researchers to explore different dimensions of the area, develop various multidisciplinary collaborative studies, and broaden the scope of research state.

### 7.4.5 Keyword Statistics

Figure 7.6 shows the keyword statistics map on author keywords. A total of 581 keywords were identified from the extracted datasheet. Keyword statistics measure the word's frequency and analyzes the importance of a term in a text (Egbert & Biber, 2019; Zhao et al., 2020). The researcher segregated the keywords based on the frequency of occurrence. A threshold limit of five was set, which led to the identification of nine keywords. The extracted map shows that the machine learning application is gaining momentum and research studies are being developed.

Still, there is scarcity of studies in the area, thus, upcoming researchers should consider the keyword statistics and develop research studies that broaden the scope of the research fraternity. Table 7.1 identifies the keyword statistics, including total link strength and frequency of use. It provides an idea for upcoming research to identify the research strengths as well to develop research studies for understanding the application and benefits of machine learning for predicting mental disorders among elderly patients as well as providing solutions to manage with effective measures.

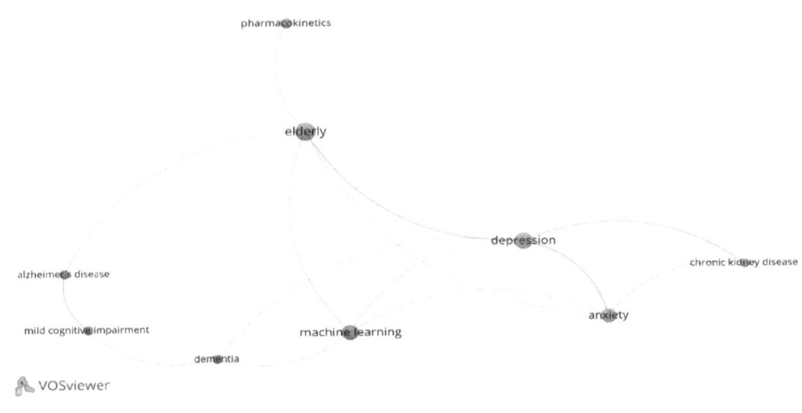


**Figure 7.6**  Keyword statistics.

**Table 7.1** Keyword Linkage

| S. NO | KEYWORD | OCCURRENCES | TOTAL LINK STRENGTH |
| --- | --- | --- | --- |
| 1 | Depression | 16 | 17 |
| 2 | Anxiety | 12 | 10 |
| 3 | Elderly | 19 | 9 |
| 4 | Chronic kidney diseases | 5 | 6 |
| 5 | Machine learning | 14 | 4 |
| 6 | Alzheimer disease | 5 | 4 |
| 7 | Dementia | 5 | 3 |
| 8 | Mild Cognitive Impairment | 7 | 3 |
| 9 | Pharmacokinetics | 5 | 3 |
| 10 | Lidocaine | 5 | 0 |

### 7.4.6 *Citation Analysis*

Citation analysis identifies the highly cited articles in the area of machine learning for predicting mental disorders. It evaluates how frequently other articles cite a specific study and recognizes the standing and effect in the concerned field (Kumar et al., 2020). The present research analyzed the citation of 189 articles. The research constrained the threshold limit to ten; it signifies a study must have cited at least ten times to be included in the analysis. Although 94 articles were outlined for subsequent analysis in the study, only those articles that establish strong links were considered and presents in Figure 7.7. Four articles had maximum citations.

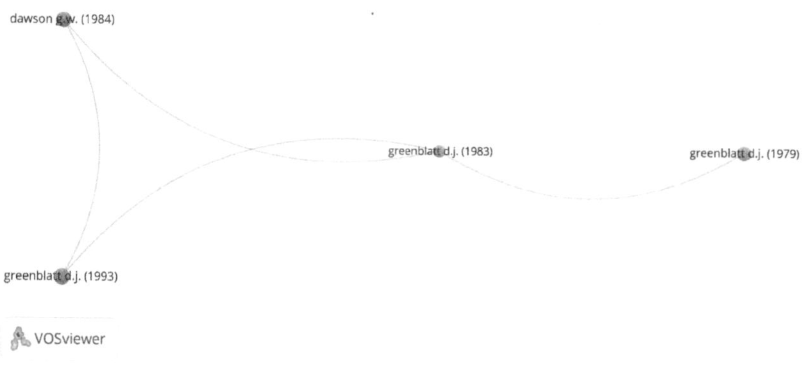


**Figure 7.7** Citation analysis.

Taking the top-cited articles into account, it can be determined that these articles provide a pragmatic and theoretical clarity toward understanding the importance, benefits, and different elements of machine learning for predicting disorders and providing more measures and solutions for improving the conditions among elderly patients.

### 7.4.7 Co-citation Analysis

Co-citation analysis aims to understand the most influential research study and map the intellectual structure in the area (Park & Shea, 2020). The research work executes co-citation analysis to identify the connection among the 189 extracted articles from the Scopus database. The set threshold limit was 20 to be included in the analysis and 44 sources meet the set criterion. Figure 7.8 shows the identified results. *NeuroImage* is the highly considered journal with a total of 113 citations. Other journals like *Neurology* and *The Lancet* are the next journals with maximum citations. Thus, the co-citation analysis signifies that these are the few journals with maximum citations. Identifying the journals provides a noteworthy idea regarding existing studies as well as gaps that exist in the literature. Therefore, the co-citation analysis provides an idea on identifying the journal's statistics to gain an idea for the most appropriate journal for publishing research studies by upcoming researchers. In addition, co-citation can help identify more journals from multidisciplinary sources to broaden the scope of the topic in every field.

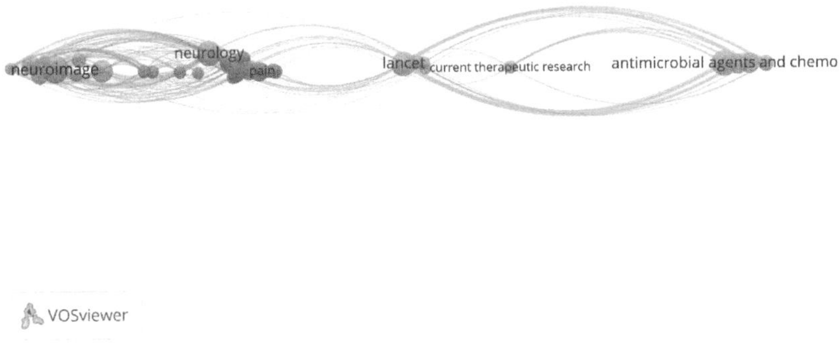


**Figure 7.8**   Co-citation analysis.

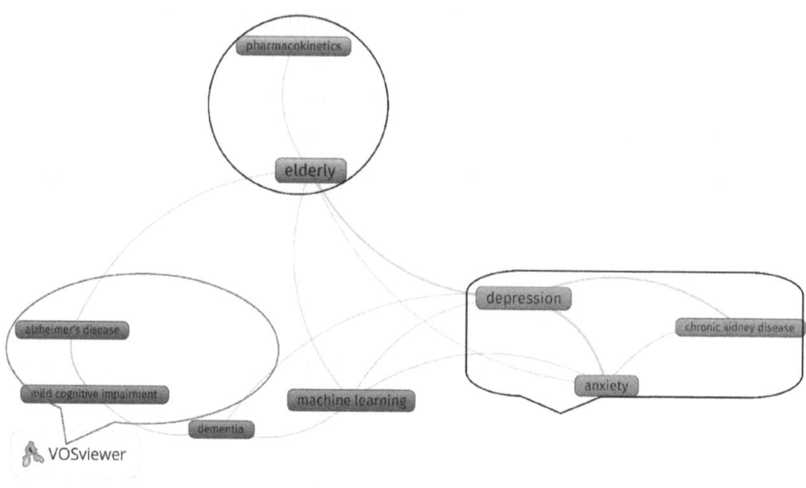


**Figure 7.9**   Thematic area identification.

### 7.4.8 Thematic Areas Identification

The discussion on keyword occurrence led to the identification of thematic areas. The analysis led to the formulation of three clusters. The clusters are named and denoted by using different colors and shapes. The clusters are "Machine learning and mental disorders," "Machine learning and Pharmacokinetics," and "Machine learning and cognitive impairment." Figure 7.9 shows the identified clusters in machine learning applications in predicting mental disorders among elderly patients. In continuation, the researcher conducted a deep analysis of existing research studies in the developed thematic areas to frame the future research questions for upcoming researchers.

Table 7.2 identifies the relationship between developed clusters and keywords associated with them. It signifies the researcher understands the existing studies in a particular keyword and established relationship with future studies.

**Table 7.2**   Groups Based on Keywords

| S. NO | GROUP | NAME OF THE GROUP | KEYWORDS |
|---|---|---|---|
| 1 | Group one | Machine learning and mental disorders | Depression, anxiety, and chronic kidney disease |
| 2 | Group two | Machine learning and pharmacokinetics | Pharmacokinetics |
| 3 | Group three | Machine learning and cognitive impairment | Dementia, Alzheimer disease |

*7.4.8.1 Machine Learning and Mental Disorders*   Bdozk and Lindenberg (2018) discussed that data derived from patients can enable the development of better treatment options. Machine learning allows the development of custom information, measurable and observable that can easily predict disease for early treatment. The study by Shatte et al. (2019) explained the required data for developing various treatment measures that can address disorders and problems through different techniques such as neural networks, support vector machines and decision trees. Priya et al. (2020) used machine learning algorithms to understand and predict anxiety and depression disorders to actively develop treatment solutions and minimize the level of panic among patients. Chekroud et al. (2021) analyzed how machine learning enables the prediction of mental disorders through the use of sensors and identifies the risk at a faster pace by enabling health practitioners to develop solutions and more advanced treatment mechanisms. Though the relationship between machine learning and mental disorders is well represented in the existing literature and explained the significant role in predicting mental disorders, there are still many aspects that need to be measured. Therefore, the current discussion leads to the formulation of two research questions from the thematic area to be explored by future researchers that would aid in the understanding, analysis, and prediction of treatment solutions for mental disorders.

*7.4.8.2 Machine Learning and Pharmacokinetics*   Kumar et al. (2018) examined the relevance of machine learning models and techniques for understanding various properties such as absorption, distribution, metabolism, and exertion. In Iriarte et al. (2019), the researchers explored the severity of toxicity among patients using machine learning techniques. On the other hand, Wang et al. (2020) measured different pharmacokinetic properties using deep learning and machine learning algorithms to obtain optimized solutions. Miljkovic et al. (2021) explored the potentialities of machine learning models in drug discovery, which has a lasting impact on decision-making related to drug-discovery projects. Chou and Lin (2022) discussed integrating machine learning techniques for developing different physiologically based pharmacokinetic models for drug development and the assessment of risk in chemicals. Through these previously mentioned studies, it has been identified that machine learning techniques have been prominently adopted in pharmacokinetics for decision-making, risk assessment, and predicting properties of chemicals and toxicity (Oyaga-Iriarte et al. 2019), but many other features and characteristics still need to be examined (Zisberg 2017). Therefore, the existing discussion led to the formulation of two research questions from the thematic area to be explored by future researchers, which enable the understanding, analysis, and prediction of the interpretability of factors and characteristics in pharmacokinetics.

*7.4.8.3 Machine Learning and Cognitive Impairment*   Pellegrini et al. (2018) analyzed the role of machine learning in measuring neuroimaging cognitive disorders. It systematically provided tools to understand risk and develop robust clinical trials. Research by Taheri Gorji and Kaabouch (2019) and Spasov et al. (2019) stated that machine relations provide the scope to distinguish between healthy people and mild cognitive impairment using magnetic imaging resonance results. Stamate et al. (2020) developed multilayer perceptron models that predicted cognitive impairment and considered time-related information as a close factor for treatment solutions. Further, the studies by Ansart et al. (2021), Sakatani and Yener (2022), and Javed et al. (2021) discussed that machine learning, through good practices, can be considered as a tool for decision support systems for identifying cognitive impairment and proposing treatment solutions. Following those studies, Mirzaei and Adeli (2022) discussed machine learning algorithms such as support vector machines, random forest, and convolutional neural networks as promising tools that can transfer relevant information for better treatment and results (Byrne & Pachana 2010). Though the relationship between machine learning and cognitive impairment is well represented in the existing literature and explained the significant role in predicting diseases, there are many aspects that still need to be identified, as many powerful algorithms have been recently developed such as the neural network, neural dynamic classification algorithm, and finite element machine for fast learning (Bokma et al., 2022). Thus, the existing discussion led to the formulation of two research questions from the thematic area to be explored by future researchers, which enable the understanding, analysis, and prediction of treatment solutions for cognitive impairment diseases.

**Table 7.3**  Outlined Future Research Questions

| THEMATIC AREAS | FUTURE RESEARCH QUESTIONS |
| --- | --- |
| Machine learning and mental disorders | "What is the role of machine learning to handle mental disorders effectively?"<br>"How do we develop predictive models using machine learning for proper risk assessment?" |
| Machine learning and pharmacokinetics | "How does machine learning improve decision-making and risk assessment in different aspects of pharmacokinetics?"<br>"How do we measure the interpretability and efficiency of developed models in pharmacokinetics?" |
| Machine learning and cognitive impairment | "What is the role of machine learning algorithms for developing effective methods of detection in cognitive impairment?"<br>"What is the impact of machine learning in the health sector on predicting, understanding, and treating cognitive impairment patients in a shorter time period?" |

*7.4.8.4 Outlined Future Research Questions* Upcoming researchers should consider and examine the probable relationships through the developed research questions and add value to the existing literature from a new perspective. This aids the government, health practitioners, and specialists in assessing the benefits of its application as well as enhances long-run performance. Thus, future developed questions give opportunities to researchers to contribute to the impending research agenda through value addition to the health sector, research, and academic fraternity in Table 7.3.

## 7.5  Implications of the Study

### 7.5.1  Practical Implications

With the change in time, environment, and technological conditions, people are encountering multiple challenges. Mental stability is an important aspect specifically among elderly people. The implementation of improved and modern practices can play a substantial role in managing mental disorders as well as improving mental conditions. Thus, machine learning in predicting anxiety and depression disorders at an early stage among elderly patients can aid in develop treatment measures that will prove better and more effective. This study attempts to examine the role of machine learning from preceding studies and also develop network maps to explore the relevant contributions through authors and keywords statistics in the field. The current study would help explain the theoretical aspects of the application of machine learning in developing different predictive models that will synthesize different treatment solutions through the decision tree and neural network, creating a modern approach for elderly patients. The study also analyzed the brief usage of machine learning for providing customized and patient-friendly services for better results.

### 7.5.2 *Social Implications*

The present study conducted a review and bibliometric analysis to understand the link between the application of machine learning in predicting mental disorders such as anxiety and depression among elderly patients at an early stage for better treatment. Changing societal conditions and the isolation of part of the population are predictors of mental disorders among elderly patients. Though studies were developed to understand the mental disorders among elderly patients, every research expressed a new approach to developing treatment. Thus, the present research collaborated with the existing studies and developed a composite work to understand the relevance of technological changes and how they can be implemented in the health sector for better results. Predicting anxiety and depression among elderly patients at an early stage with accurate and valid information can enable them to lead a stress-free and healthy life, which enhances their social relationships as well as their relationships with family while also efficiently screening for depression.

### 7.6 Discussion

The ultimate explanations of this study indicated that the technique is gaining momentum and has expanded to every field including the health sector, but there are many more facets to be uncovered. The developed research questions of the study identified the source with the maximum publication of papers on machine learning: the journal *BMJ Open, which* belongs to the British Medical Association.

The yearly trend analysis shows an increase, specifically in 2020, in interest among the academic fraternity. The application of machine learning is fascinating and gaining attention from upcoming researchers and has led to the replacement of traditional treatment solutions with more modern methods. The research provides insight to understand past, present, and future perspectives in machine learning. It also provides insight into prolific authors and countries as well as into network maps on author/co-authorship, keyword statistics, citation, and co-citation information. Further, it led to the identification of three major thematic areas and developed a future framework for upcoming researchers. The research streams are machine learning and mental disorders, machine learning and pharmacokinetics, and machine learning and cognitive impairment. Based on the above discussions, the proposed framework in Figure 7.10 aims to identify the features, and components for effective implementation of machine learning. Further, the upcoming researcher needs to evaluate and assess the relative prominence of the framework stages to be implemented and verified in machine learning applications.

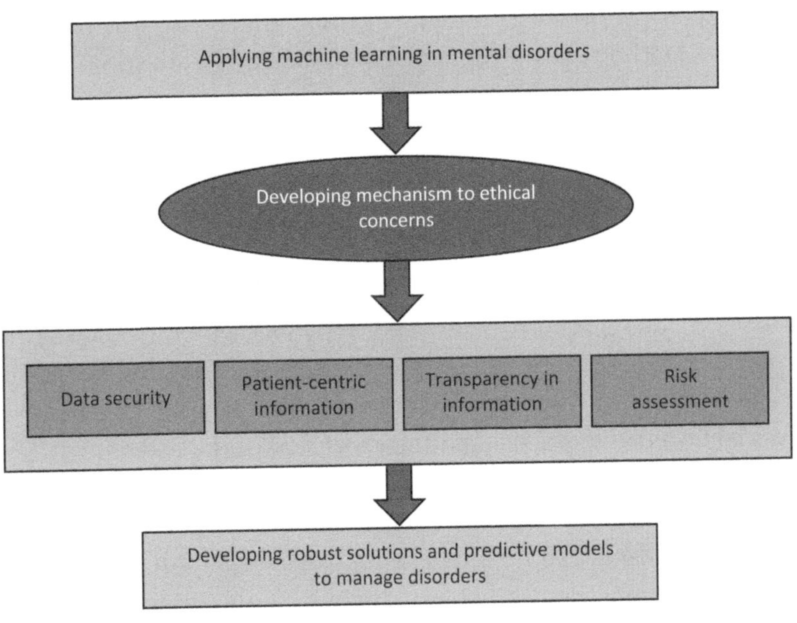


**Figure 7.10**    An integrative framework to measure the application of machine learning.

## 7.7 Conclusion and Future Scope of the Research

The present research has a few limitations that can be addressed and considered by future researchers despite the previous discussion. First, the application of machine learning in the health sector is in its early stages, not only predicting mental disorders but also developing required solutions to various diseases, and is highly essential, requiring a thorough research-oriented approach. Second, only the Scopus database has been considered for searching papers, whereas other databases like PubMed and Web of Science can be considered to develop a comparative approach and analyze the results. Considering the cited point in future studies, other repositories can be examined for identifying data for conducting similar studies. Third, the research focuses on presenting a broader view for future researchers by conducting studies that add value to the domain. Hence, the extracted results can consider the changes and incorporate new aspects in forthcoming studies and compare the results. Considering the previously mentioned limitations, future studies can be developed. However, the present research is an amalgamated bibliometric study that provides a route for future researchers to develop empirically tested models and applications and attempt theory verification. Further, this study was based on a single method, i.e., SLR and bibliometric visualization. Future researchers may extend their work on the meta-analysis approach to identify the application of the technique in other fields, rationalizing the results of this research and justifying the generalizability of the proposed techniques and concepts

This research is a step toward understanding the benefits of the application of machine learning in predicting anxiety and depression disorders among aged patients. The study focused on measuring the current state of research in machine learning applications in handling mental disorders. The research through bibliometric visualization was approached to understand the expansion of the technique. Thus, machine learning has expanded into every sector including the health sector. The study developed different thematic areas, determining how machine learning can be integrated for mental disorders prediction, cognitive impairment, and pharmacokinetics. The study analyzed the research state in terms of contributors, keyword statistics, citation, and co-citation analysis and developed an integrative framework for impending researchers to explore the application of machine learning and take the study as a benchmark for understanding the present and minimizing the gaps for achieving better results and performance.

# References


Ali, S., & Azhar, N. (2022). Old Age People Emotional Stress Prediction During Outbreak Using Machine Learning Methods. In *Predictive Analytics of Psychological Disorders in Healthcare: Data Analytics on Psychological Disorders*, 177–196). Singapore: Springer Nature Singapore.

Andrews, J. A. (2018). *Applying digital technology to the prediction of depression and anxiety in older adults* (Doctoral dissertation, University of Sheffield).

Ansart, M., Epelbaum, S., Bassignana, G., Bône, A., Bottani, S., Cattai, T., & Durrleman, S. (2021). Predicting the progression of mild cognitive impairment using machine learning: a systematic, quantitative and critical review. *Medical Image Analysis*, *67*, 101848.

Bhatnagar, S., Agarwal, J., & Sharma, O. R. (2023). Detection and classification of anxiety in university students through the application of machine learning. *Procedia Computer Science*, *218*, 1542–1550.

Bokma, W. A., Zhutovsky, P., Giltay, E. J., Schoevers, R. A., Penninx, B. W., Van Balkom, A. L., & Van Wingen, G. A. (2022). Predicting the naturalistic course in anxiety disorders using clinical and biological markers: a machine learning approach. *Psychological Medicine*, *52*(1), 57–67.

Byrne, G. J., & Pachana, N. A. (2010). Anxiety and depression in the elderly: do we know any more. *Current Opinion in Psychiatry*, *23*(6), 504–509.

Bzdok, D., & Lindenberg, A.M. (2018). Machine learning for precision psychiatry: opportunities and challenges. *Biological Psychiatry: Cognitive Neuroscience and Neuroimaging 3*(3), 223–230, DOI: https://doi.org/10.1016/j.bpsc.2017.11.007

Chekroud, A. M., Bondar, J., Delgadillo, J., Doherty, G., Wasil, A., Fokkema, M., & Choi, K. (2021). The promise of machine learning in predicting treatment outcomes in psychiatry. *World Psychiatry*, *20*(2), 154–170.

Chou, W. C., & Lin, Z. (2022). Machine learning and artificial intelligence in physiologically based pharmacokinetic modeling. *Toxicological Sciences*, *191*(1), 1–14.

Egbert, J., & Biber, D. (2019). Incorporating text dispersion into keyword analyses. *Corpora*, *14*(1), 77–104.

Gerard J.B & Nancy A.P. (2010). Development and validation of a short form of the Geriatric Anxiety Inventory- the GAI-SF. *International Psychogeiatrics*, *23*(1), 125–131.

Hatton, C. M., Paton, L. W., McMillan, D., Cussens, J., Gilbody, S., & Tiffin, P. A. (2019). Predicting persistent depressive symptoms in older adults: a machine learning approach to personalised mental healthcare. *Journal of Affective Disorders, 246*, 857–860.

Iriarte, J., Elliott, S., Maezumi, S. Y., Alves, D., Gonda, R., Robinson, M., Souza, J.G.d., Watling, J., & Handley, J. (2019). The origins of Amazonian landscapes: Plant cultivation, domestication and the spread of food production in tropical South America. *Quanternary Science Reviews* 248, 106582, DOI: https://doi.org/10.1016/j.quascirev.2020.106582

Islam, F., Wang, J., Farooq, M.A., Khan, M.S.S., Xu, L., Zhu, J., Zhao, M., Muños, S., Li, Q.X., & Zhou, W. (2018). Potential impact of the herbicide 2,4-dichlorophenoxyacetic acid on human and ecosystems, *Environment International*, 111. DOI: 10.1016/j.envint.2017.10.020

Javed, A. R., Fahad, L. G., Farhan, A. A., Abbas, S., Srivastava, G., Parizi, R. M., & Khan, M. S. (2021). Automated cognitive health assessment in smart homes using machine learning. *Sustainable Cities and Society, 65*, 102572.

Kumar, P., Garg, S., & Garg, A. (2020). Assessment of anxiety, depression and stress using machine learning models. *Procedia Computer Science, 171*, 1989–1998.

Kumar, R., Sharma, A., Siddiqui, M. H., & Tiwari, R. K. (2018). Promises of machine learning approaches in prediction of absorption of compounds. *Mini Reviews in Medicinal Chemistry, 18*(3), 196–207.

Kumar, S. (2015). "Co-authorship networks: a review of the literature. *Aslib Journal of Information Management, 67*(1), 55–73.

Kunze, K. N., Polce, E. M., Rasio, J., & Nho, S. J. (2021). Machine learning algorithms predict clinically significant improvements in satisfaction after hip arthroscopy. *Arthroscopy: The Journal of Arthroscopic & Related Surgery, 37*(4), 1143–1151.

Kunze, K. N., Polce, E. M., Rasio, J., & Nho, S. J. (2021). Machine learning algorithms predict clinically significant improvements in satisfaction after hip arthroscopy. *Arthroscopy: The Journal of Arthroscopic & Related Surgery, 37*(4), 1143–1151.

Meester J. A. N., Verstraeten A., Schepers D., Alaerts M., Laer L. V., & Loyes B. L. (2017). Differences in manifestations of Marfan syndrome, Ehlers-Danlos syndrome, and Loeys-Dietz syndrome. *Annals of Cardiothoracic Surgery, 6*(6), 582–594.

Miljković, F., Martinsson, A., Obrezanova, O., Williamson, B., Johnson, M., Sykes, A., & Greene, N. (2021). Machine learning models for human in vivo pharmacokinetic parameters with in-house validation. *Molecular Pharmaceutics, 18*(12), 4520–4530.

Mirzaei, G., & Adeli, H. (2022). Machine learning techniques for diagnosis of alzheimer disease, mild cognitive disorder, and other types of dementia. *Biomedical Signal Processing and Control, 72*, 103293.

Mohr, D. C., Zhang, M., & Schueller, S. M. (2017). Personal sensing: understanding mental health using ubiquitous sensors and machine learning. *Annual Review of Clinical Psychology, 13*, 23.

Montoya R. M., Kershaw C., & Prosser J. L. (2018). A meta-analytic investigation of the relation between interpersonal attraction and enacted behavior. *Psychological Bulletin*, 144(7), 673–709.

Nemesure, M. D., Heinz, M. V., Huang, R., & Jacobson, N. C. (2021). Predictive modeling of depression and anxiety using electronic health records and a novel machine learning approach with artificial intelligence. *Scientific Reports*, *11*(1), 1–9.

Oyaga-Iriarte, E., Insausti, A., Sayar, O., & Aldaz, A. (2019). Prediction of irinotecan toxicity in metastatic colorectal cancer patients based on machine learning models with pharmacokinetic parameters. *Journal of Pharmacological Sciences*, *140*(1), 20–25.

Pandit, M., Azwaan, M., Wani, S., Ibrahim, A. A., Abdulghafor, R. A. A., & Gulzar, Y. (2023). Examining factors for anxiety and depression prediction. *International Journal on Perceptive and Cognitive Computing*, *9*(1), 70–79.

Park, H., & Shea, P. (2020). A review of ten-year research through co-citation analysis: online learning, distance learning, and blended learning. *Online Learning*, *24*(2), 225–244.

Pellegrini, E., Ballerini, L., Hernandez, M. D. C. V., Chappell, F. M., González-Castro, V., Anblagan, D., & Wardlaw, J. M. (2018). Machine learning of neuroimaging for assisted diagnosis of cognitive impairment and dementia: a systematic review. *Alzheimer's & Dementia: Diagnosis, Assessment & Disease Monitoring*, *10*, 519–535.

Pickering, C., & Byrne, J. (2014). "The benefits of publishing systematic quantitative literature reviews for PhD candidates and other early-career researchers. *Higher Education Research and Development*, *33*(3), 534–548.

Priya, A., Garg, S., & Tigga, N. P. (2020). Predicting anxiety, depression and stress in modern life using machine learning algorithms. *Procedia Computer Science*, *167*, 1258–1267.

Rajawat, A.S., Bedi, P., Goyal, S.B., Shukla, P.K., Zaguia, A., Jain, A., & Khan, M.M. (2021). "Reformist framework for improving human security for mobile robots in indutry 4.0". *Mobile Information Systems*, 2021 (1), Article ID: 4744220, 10 pages, DOI: https://doi.org/10.1155/2021/4744220.

Sakatani, K., & Yener, G. (2022). Application of machine learning in the diagnosis of dementia. *Frontiers in Neurology*, *13*, 860607.

Saraçlı, Ö., Akca, A. S. D., Atasoy, N., Önder, Ö., Şenormancı, Ö., Kaygısız, İsmet., & Atik, L. (2015). The relationship between quality of life and cognitive functions, anxiety and depression among hospitalized elderly patients. *Clinical Psychopharmacology and Neuroscience*, *13*(2), 194.

Shatte, A. B., Hutchinson, D. M., & Teague, S. J. (2019). Machine learning in mental health: a scoping review of methods and applications. *Psychological Medicine*, *49*(9), 1426–1448.

Shinde, S. A., & Rajeswari, P. R. (2018). Intelligent health risk prediction systems using machine learning: a review. *International Journal of Engineering & Technology*, *7*(3), 1019–1023.

Spasov, S., Passamonti, L., Duggento, A., Lio, P., & Toschi, N. Alzheimer's Disease Neuroimaging Initiative (2019). A parameter-efficient deep learning approach to predict conversion from mild cognitive impairment to Alzheimer's disease. *Neuroimage, 189,* 276–287.

Stamate, D., Smith, R., Tsygancov, R., Vorobev, R., Langham, J., Stahl, D., & Reeves, D. (2020, June). Applying deep learning to predicting dementia and mild cognitive impairment. In *IFIP international conference on artificial intelligence applications and innovations* (308–319). Springer, Cham.

Su, F., Xu, S., Sayer, E.J., Chen, W., Du, Y., & Lu, X. (2021). "Distinct storage mechanisms of soil organic carbon in coniferous forest and evergreen broadleaf forest in tropical China", *Journal of Environmental Management* 295, 113142. DOI: https://doi.org/10.1016/j.jenvman.2021.113142

Taheri Gorji, H., & Kaabouch, N. (2019). A deep learning approach for diagnosis of mild cognitive impairment based on MRI images. *Brain Sciences, 9*(9), 217.

Tranfield, D., Denyer, D., & Smart, P. (2003). "Towards a methodology for developing evidence informed management knowledge by means of systematic review. *British Journal of Management, 14*(3), 207–222.

Trevisani, M., & Tuzzi, A. (2015). A portrait of JASA: the history of statistics through analysis of keyword counts in an early scientific journal. *Quality & Quantity, 49*(3), 1287–1304.

van Eeden, W. A., Luo, C., van Hemert, A. M., Carlier, I. V., Penninx, B. W., Wardenaar, K. J., & Giltay, E. J. (2021). Predicting the 9-year course of mood and anxiety disorders with automated machine learning: a comparison between auto-sklearn, naïve Bayes classifier, and traditional logistic regression. *Psychiatry Research, 299,* 113823.

Wang, R., Liu, Y., Lu, Y., Zhang, J., Liu, P., Yao, Y., & Grekousis, G. (2019). Perceptions of built environment and health outcomes for older Chinese in Beijing: a big data approach with Street view images and deep learning technique. *Computers, Environment and Urban Systems, 78,* 101386.

Wang, X., Liu, M., Zhang, L., Wang, Y., Li, Y., & Lu, T. (2020). Optimizing pharmacokinetic property prediction based on integrated datasets and a deep learning approach. *Journal of Chemical Information and Modeling, 60*(10), 4603–4613.

Zhao, Y., Cheng, S., Yu, X., & Xu, H. (2020). Chinese public's attention to the COVID-19 epidemic on social media: observational descriptive study. *Journal of Medical Internet Research, 22*(5), e18825.

Zisberg, A. (2017). Anxiety and depression in older patients: the role of culture and acculturation. *International Journal for Equity in Health, 16*(1), 1–10.

# Index